Secrets of a SKINNY JEAN QUEEN ®

A 7-STEP GUIDE TO HELP YOU EAT & ACT LIKE YOU HAVE SOME SENSE

CAROLYN GRAY

Printed in the United States of America

Carolyn Gray International, LLC
5746 Union Mill Road, PMB 495
Clifton, Virginia 20124

Cover Photo: Donald Harvey
Cover Concept: Kristen Argonis

ISBN: 0-9665171-4-8
ISBN-13: 9780966517149
Library of Congress Control Number: 2009905271

Visit www.carolyngrayinternational.com to order additional copies.

~⌒~

Publisher's Note

The intent of this book is to present the author's ideas and perceptions about getting to a healthy weight and staying there. Although this book offers a commonsense, moderate approach to exercise and eating, **the author is not a licensed health professional, nutritionist, or a personal trainer**, and she *does not claim to have the best plan for every person's body. The advice and recommendations in this book are strictly a reflection of the author's opinions, views, and experiences, as well as her observations and research.* There are no guarantees that you will experience the same results as the author or other readers in their efforts/successes where weight loss and maintenance are concerned. *Only you and/or your physician can determine the best diet and exercise regimen for you based on your current weight, body type, physical condition, and medical history.* As a result, you have the right to disagree with the views and opinions of the author. More importantly, before you begin this or any exercise regimen, consult with your personal physician to make sure there are no pre-existing conditions that preclude an increase in physical activity.

Dedication

From my own personal experiences in trying to lose weight, I know how hard it can be to lose just five or ten pounds, so I know the challenge of trying to lose twenty, thirty, fifty pounds or more can seem overwhelming. I can only imagine the hurt and frustration that those who have serious struggles with their weight can experience. From comments/insults to stares, whispers, laughter, or something as subtle as a stranger not bothering to make eye contact... Without realizing it or intending to, as people, we can be so mean to each other.

I really don't believe people realize how hurtful their words and looks can be to someone who may already be suffering from insecurities or sensitivities about his or her weight. One cruel joke about a person's weight or a judgmental look can negatively affect someone's life forever, undermining self-esteem and stealing hope... For this reason, I dedicate this book as an offer of help and encouragement to anyone who has ever struggled with weight. It is my prayer that this book will help readers reach whatever weight loss goals they may have because I know it can be done, and I believe that anyone who wants to can do it!

Acknowledgments

First, I must give thanks to the Lord for giving me the ability to write and for allowing me to go through the challenges and trials that I have so that I have the material needed to write a book such as this. Mostly I thank Him for grace and mercy.

I also owe my husband a world of thanks for being my friend and for giving me the love, support, and freedom to do the things that I want to do, such as writing books that publishers may not be beating down my door to get.

I need to thank my sons as well. I love them more than I thought it was possible to love anyone, and without my realizing it, their very existence always makes me want to do and be better. This puts a lot of wind beneath a mom's wings.

My mother also deserves my sincerest thanks for the strong hand that kept me on the straight and narrow as I passed through environments that held a lot of pitfalls for me. *Without her I wouldn't be the woman I am today.*

This is the point where some may think I am crazy, but there are a few more abstract people/groups to thank (*reading the book will help you understand why*):

- *Upward Bound*—a program for economically disadvantaged high school students that helped me see beyond my life in the projects and put me on a path towards college. The stipends over the summer, field trips and college-prep classes were a tremendous blessing.

- *E. I. DuPont and the Savannah River Plant*—a company that reached out to high school students with technical internships during the '80s. They were looking for high school seniors at my school, but for some reason they accepted me even though I was a junior. I interned with them for three summers in computer science, and it made a huge difference in my life and career in terms of money for college and career experience when I graduated.
- *Georgia-Pacific*—the company that helped me accomplish my very first big goal–a college degree. The check that was there waiting for me every semester was the foundation/safety net that helped finance my education.
- *My "Angel" at Clemson (Dr. Arthur Pellerin)*—the computer science professor who threw me a much-needed lifeline in the midst of changing my major during the last leg of my college career. *Without his help, I would not have my degree.*
- *Starbucks*—the perfect writing environment (the *Cheers* of the twenty-first century) with its friendly staff, good music, refreshing ethos water, and their delicious *Signature Hot Chocolate*. It is my all-time favorite place to write, and it is where I overcame the writer's block and distractions that prevented me from finishing this book. It is a haven for anyone with creative aspirations—where strangers meet, exchange ideas and become friends. Starbucks customers even inspired and encouraged me during the final stages of this book. *For all of this I am truly grateful.*

Contents

~

Prologue

Sssshhhh.... *Not while I'm thinking...* I am trying *so* very hard to still my busy, busy mind and reach some sort of mental nirvana, *if it is possible...* A faraway, tranquil, and quiet place where my thoughts are not running a mile a minute, where I am not totally absorbed, overwhelmed, or frozen like a deer in the headlights by a never-ending to-do list that seems to grow exponentially as I desperately struggle to juggle my many personas—wife, mom, writer, husband's assistant in business, entrepreneur, IT consultant, *person, etc...* I don't know about anyone else, but I find it extremely difficult to keep all of the "balls" in the air, which makes me wonder *why* is it that I am always finding new tasks to do or think about? I am sometimes so stressed, *all of my own doing,* that I struggle to live in the moment and enjoy the happiness I have been blessed with and so easily take for granted.

However, during the rare times that I can finally get my mind to be still and quiet, something truly spectacular happens. I am finally able to see the *true, lasting,* and *wonderful* blessings that are present in my life **right now**, not what I want or am trying to achieve, but *what I already have* and *what matters most*. I can see it all in my mind, but now it is in 3-D, with surround sound, on the 108-inch high-definition plasma screen in my mind... I see *quality of life*—the love of my family, our health, my marriage, lots of laughter, time spent together, peace... These precious moments of reflection are indeed a beautiful wake-up call.

Why is it though that I never take the time to appreciate these things until *after* I have fussed at my children for the hundredth time about *trivial trivialities* such as: turning off the lights in the bathroom, not throwing clothes/toys on the floor, remembering to wash their hands after using the restroom, not yelling at each other (*even though I am often yelling when I tell them*), blah, blah, blah, etc., etc...

Amazingly enough, after I take a few deep breaths, my youngest son often reminds me to do this by saying "*breathe*" or "*chill*" *Mombo* (*his occasional pet name for me, which I find wonderfully endearing, and it makes me want to give him the biggest hug and kiss...if only he'd let me without squirming or running away*) I force myself to mentally break free from the crazy whirlwind that has become my life (e.g., work, cooking, cleaning, chauffeuring kids to practices/games/activities, etc.). It is during these moments that I privately enjoy the loveliest, happiest, and yummiest thoughts of my husband and children. They don't know it, but I am often amazed that *they are really mine*—the close-knit, loving, ever-laughing, often pain-in-the-butt/uptight/arguing-over-nonsense, *wouldn't-trade-em-for-the-world family* I always dreamt of having. However, sometimes I forget how wonderful they are and how fortunate I am to have them, and if you ever see me staring off into space and smiling to myself, this is what I am probably thinking...

It is during these sweet, brief moments that my sons may look at me as if I am crazy because I am usually staring at their faces without saying anything... My smile is often distant as I drink in the *beauty* of their faces, the *softness* of their hands and the warmth of their scent... *Hmmmm....* It is almost as if I am breathing them in, and I feel so very *thankful. Truly grateful. Blissfully happy in that moment...* And most of all, *blessed beyond measure.* Even though my life is far from perfect, these moments of reflection help me to see how much I have to be thankful, grateful, and happy about: my relationship with God and my family; the health of my body and the members of my family; my marriage—over eighteen years and going strong; and too many material comforts, opportunities, and resources to name... *All things that I could only dream of as a teenager growing up in the projects of Augusta, Georgia...*

~

Chapter 1

I n t r o d u c t i o n

It has been said, and I agree, that the definition of insanity is *doing the same thing over and over again and expecting a different result*. However, many of us perfectly *sane* people continue to live and eat the same way year after year, yet we hope and pray for different results in our body and health (*I know I used to, and sometimes still do*). How *insane* is that? One of the main goals of this book is to offer ideas and new ways of thinking to help you start doing some things differently today so you can get the results you want in the future.

Believe it or not, this is the heart of my so-called *diet* secret—based on the results I see in my body and my life, I make changes in my food intake/choices, my thinking, my physical activities and/or my life's focus until I get the results that I want. Doing this has helped me to stay the same size for almost twenty years (a size 6, *the right size for me, but not necessarily the right size for you*). I may put on a few pounds, but I always find my way back, even after having children—*without dieting or going to the gym on a regular basis*. When people ask my "*secret*," I want to tell them, but I realize that a good bit of explanation is required before my methods (*or my madness*) can be easily understood or applied to someone else's life. So this is my attempt to condense twenty years' worth of life-lessons into tangible advice that can be used by anyone. I share examples from my life, including mistakes I have made and recovered from, as well as the regrouping I still do from time to time. As you read this book, you will be given opportunities to analyze areas of your life and apply principles/tips as they make sense. I truly believe this will put you on a path to making the gradual changes that will add up to major differences in your life, body (i.e., weight and fitness), and health.

I must admit that it is such a blessing to be in better physical shape now, at forty-three, than I was at eighteen—*slimmer and more fit than I was before I had children*. Sometimes it is hard for me to believe, but I pretty much feel the same as I did at twenty-five (except for occasional knee, hip, and shoulder pain when I do too much or don't stretch). This has led me to the conclusion that age really is nothing but a number. This was a very freeing epiphany, especially as I remember having so many preconceived ideas of how forty-, fifty-, and sixty-year-olds look, act and feel. I am sure you may have too, but I am here to tell you that we can look as good and as healthy as we want to look regardless of our age!

It is comical now, but I remember thinking as a kid that to be a grandmother you had to be overweight. Can you believe that? I think this stemmed from the fact that almost every kid I knew as a child had a grandmother that was overweight. Now that I am older and wiser, I realize that just because we get older and our metabolisms slow down, it doesn't mean we *have* to gain large amounts of weight. In fact, just by using a few of the tips found in this book you can ensure that you don't. However, if you *let* yourself believe that weight gain and aging go hand in hand, you will probably gain excess weight, but you don't "*have to.*"

What if as we age and gain more wisdom, we start and/or continue to be active and eat what we like in moderation? Wouldn't that counteract some of the damage caused by age? *I think so.* Even though coronary heart disease is the number one killer in the United States (*according to the American Heart Association*), we don't *have to* get it. The same is true with diabetes and hypertension, we don't "*have to*"get these diseases. We may, but for the most part preventative measures can keep many of us from being affected by these potentially life-threatening diseases. The question then becomes are you willing to take a long, hard look at how you are living today, and make small changes, as needed, to live a better life tomorrow? I truly hope you are. *I know I am!*

As you read further, you will find practical, *get-started-today* tips on how to find out what ails you on an emotional/mental level (*what drives you to overeat*) and move beyond it, how to get help, get moving, and learn how to really *eat like you have some sense*. I am sure you are wondering how on earth I came up with the concept of *"eating like you have some sense."* Well, as a kid growing up in South Carolina and Georgia, I heard my share of crazy expressions from adults such as: "Go somewhere and sit down, and *act like you have some sense,"* or *"Stop running around acting like you don't have any sense!"* It was beyond me how one acts like they have some sense. I didn't have a clue what that meant, but out of fear of punishment, I learned *real quick* that it meant to immediately stop indulging in whatever foolishness I was engaging in, or I would suffer, *and I do mean suffer*, the consequences. Oddly enough, as I worked on this book, I realized that the "acting like you have some sense" ideology can be applied to weight loss and maintenance, as well as it can be to behavior. As an example, if we continue to overindulge where food is concerned, *eating like we don't have any sense*, we will suffer, *and I do mean suffer*, the possible consequences (e.g., obesity, hypertension, type 2 diabetes, heart disease, a reduced-activity lifestyle, etc.).

My goal is to help you immediately stop indulging in whatever "foolishness" you may be engaging in (*everyone has a problem area—whether it is overeating, chronic inactivity, etc.*). As a result, I will give tips on how you can learn to eat like you have some sense, so you will not suffer any of the unnecessary *consequences* I mentioned earlier. I believe the tips on eating better (*Chapter 8*) can really get you started on the right path for weight loss, but I think it is more important to work through unresolved emotional issues (*Chapter 4*), get your mind right (*Chapter 5*), and increase your physical activity (*Chapter 7*) first. You will be amazed as weight slowly starts to disappear (*the best way to achieve lasting results—weight was not gained overnight, so it will not be lost overnight*) without you even realizing it, as you are enjoying your life. The best part is that it will stay off (*as long as you continue the habits you develop, that is*).

This is what happened to me, and I have been so very thankful over the years because it was always my prayer as a child to be slim as an adult. However, because I grew up with "a little pudge," I thought my fate was to become progressively more overweight as an adult. I never knew how easy it would be to maintain a healthy weight as an adult—no diet or plan could be simpler, cheaper, more comprehensive, or as *life-changing*. I truly believe the Lord answered my prayers where my weight is concerned by giving me the revelations I am about to share with you. Maintaining my weight has been such a blessing over the years, and I believe we are blessed so that we can be a blessing to others. So it is my prayer that the information in this book will be a blessing to you as you work to reach your desired weight, *not for a week or a month*, but *for a lifetime*. As you read further it will become clear that this is not just another get-fit-quick-scheme. Instead, it is *a maintain-a-healthy-weight-for-life-plan*, and I literally cannot wait to share it with you! However, I must give you a little background on the journey that led me to this "plan" first…

~

Chapter 2

W h o ' s   T h i s   C a r o l y n   G r a y   A n d
W h y   S h o u l d   I   L i s t e n   T o   H e r ?

As new years start and end, New Year's resolutions are always at the forefront of everyone's mind. Year after year many of us put losing weight and/or getting into better shape at the top of our list. I know getting into better shape is always on mine! As obesity becomes a health issue for an increasing percentage of the American population, losing weight and/or getting into better shape should be a priority for all of us. The United States, as a whole (e.g., *White, Black, Hispanic, Indian, etc.)* has a "weight problem," and more of us are dying from illnesses such as heart disease and type 2 diabetes at younger ages, even though our quality of health care, level of education, and knowledge are the best they have ever been. This is really amazing if you think about the fact that we probably have more gyms, health/fitness clubs, exercise equipment, fitness videos, diet books, diet pills, and sugar-free, fat-free, low-fat, low-carb, low-calorie food and drinks than any other country in the world. In the land of opportunity, where we can be what we want to be, *this does not have to be our fate.*

In many cases diseases such as type 2 diabetes, hypertension and heart disease are largely preventable, especially if we can keep our weight within a *"healthy range" (see the BMI chart in Chapter 4, or check with your doctor to help determine where you are/need to be).* One of the major goals of this book is to help you reach, and keep your weight within, a "healthy range"—*not to be model-thin or to fit into a certain dress or outfit for a special occasion, and not just for a few months, but for a lifetime.* Regardless of how many times you may have dieted and failed in the past, *you can lose weight* and keep it off if you **take a good look at your life, determine where you want to be,** and *decide* **to do what it takes to get there**... This is what I did, and what I still do even today. However, if you have seen the cover, you may be asking yourself, *"What on earth does she know about a weight problem or losing weight?"* Well, I am not surprised or offended because people who only knew me after college or after having kids never *saw* the struggle. However, just because I do not have a problem now doesn't mean I never had a problem in the past... There is definitely more to me than meets the eye—*I have not always been a skinny jean queen* (someone who can fit in her favorite jeans and likes the way she looks). I *have* struggled with my weight. I *do* know what it is like not to be able to lose it, but *the good news is I know how now...* And I am ready to share *all* of the details!

~·~·~· My Story ·~·~·~

Growing up in the South, I felt there was a stigma against Black women being po' (slang *for "poor" in the scrawny sense*) or too skinny. Black women are known for having curves, but I somehow missed my fair share of the curves and got a second helping of *pudge*. So during the first half of my life I was neither po' nor slim. In fact, during my teens and very early twenties I was actually overweight. By the time I was eleven, I could wear my mother's clothes, and I often did, much to my embarrassment. The fact that this was done out of financial necessity did not make it any easier for me to accept. In fact, as you can imagine, I endured quite a bit of teasing as a result. Even though the teasing hurt, I found solace in my daydreams, where I was slim and wearing all sorts of beautiful clothes as an adult. This is probably why I tend to overdress today, wearing sundresses when others are in shorts and wearing suits and heels when others are business-casual. Of course I wanted to be slim for vanity's sake, but after seeing my grandmother die in her early sixties from type 2 diabetes-related complications, I realized I also wanted to get my weight down so diabetes would not be a part of my future.

Today, at forty-three, and after having two children (*I gained close to fifty pounds for each*), I am slimmer than I was in high school and when I went to college. I am not po', as my mother might call it, but instead of the size 11 and 13 clothes I used to wear, most of my clothes are a size 6. Although I have been advised by some family members not to lose any more weight, I feel good, and my husband and I like the way I look. So aside from a few lumps/rolls that can be smoothed out with *Spanx when I choose*, I am healthy, and so far, *Praise the Lord*, diabetes has not been an issue for me. *This is what I value most—not other people's perceptions of how I look.*

As the self-confessed queen of unsolicited advice (*I think I just like to call myself a queen*), I have found myself sharing my *secrets,* or normal eating habits, over the years with people who have asked how I consistently keep my weight within a certain range. Many of these people usually think I diet, but I don't—because *I don't believe in diets.* Why? For one, I have never had the willpower to stay on any so-called diet, and the few times I have, it didn't last long. This is mainly because I am such a picky eater, which makes it very difficult for me to stick to any prescribed eating plan. *I only want to eat what I like, not what someone recommends.* Also, many of the popular diets I see often recommend artificially-sweetened foods and drinks, which I cannot stand. The chemicals used in these products give me a headache within minutes of eating/drinking them, and I feel queasy. So if I eat or drink something sweet, *I only want it sweetened with sugar.*

As I am sure many of you can relate, the few times I have dieted, I would lose a few pounds (*usually around three*), but I would always gain them right back. Also, because I felt so deprived of my favorite foods, as soon as the diet was over, I would go crazy eating them, **and** I often wound up gaining back what I lost and more! It only took a few failed attempts for me to realize that diets are not the long-term answer for me because *I want to eat what I want to eat.* As I look around at others "trying" to diet, I realize that I am not the only one, which is one of the reasons I believe the average person does not experience long-term success with most diets.

Diets tend to be frustrating experiences, or at least they have been for me, which is why I call myself a *frustrated dieter.* Diets frustrate me to no end! I think this is due to the fact that most times, the "d" in *diet* may as well stand for "*deprivation*" or "*don't.*" *Don't* eat foods made with white flour, *don't* eat bread, *don't* eat sugar, *don't* eat dairy, *don't* eat fried foods, *don't* combine protein and carbohydrates (*how can anyone ever eat a burger, sandwich, or sub if we listen to that one?*), and the list goes on and on. When I hear some of these things I must admit the word foolishness usually comes to mind! How many people can really live in this culture and follow these types of rules, especially if foods that you really enjoy fall into these categories? *Not many.* Also, how do you explain the fact that millions of people around the world and in this country are at normal weights without being concerned with such rules and constraints?

When we feel deprived, we rebel, so one lesson I have learned is that we must find ways to still eat foods we truly enjoy, *without fear or guilt.* For me to say that I am going to live a life without sugar or white flour products (e.g., cakes, cookies, etc.) without the threat of a health risk (e.g., diabetes, etc.) **and** a doctor's strong warning would be a complete and utter waste of time *and* an absolute lie. If we are going to succeed at any weight loss plan, we must be honest and realistic with ourselves regarding what we can commit to for the long term. After battling baby-weight twice, being overwhelmed and preoccupied with family/career, aging, and seeing my metabolism slow a bit, I have learned that the way we eat to lose weight must be a moderate, consistent plan we can live with once we have reached our weight loss goal. It can't be extreme, where we skip meals, go for long periods eating very low-calorie meals or depriving ourselves of foods or snacks we enjoy. Instead, it should be a plan that regularly includes not only healthy meals, but also snacks that we enjoy so we don't walk around ready to devour everything in sight. To successfully take and keep weight off, **our lifestyle** *(i.e., our way of eating, thinking and acting)* **has to change**, *and that is what happened to me about twenty years ago…*

~·~·~· Let's Start at the Beginning ·~·~·~

People say you should never forget where you came from, but my life *back then* was so different that it sometimes feels like a large part of it was all a dream. *A bad dream…* I often joke with my husband that there are times when it seems as if I suffer from a mild form of amnesia because there are so many people and places from my past that I just cannot remember. My mother is constantly asking me if I remember this person/that person from school or my childhood who remembers me, and my usual response is, *"No, I don't remember."* And it is true, *I don't.* However, regardless of what my mind may have chosen to block out, there are some things I will never forget: *the person I was, what I wanted, what I felt, the people who loved and helped me and the invaluable lessons I learned along the way.*

As an example, I remember always wanting to be "happy" and to be a part of a loving, close-knit family that really cared about each other… I wanted to have friends that really liked me *for me,* where I was not constantly trying to fit in… I wanted not to be poor so I could go to the grocery store anytime I wanted and buy whatever I wanted without being concerned with the price (unfortunately *in my present day life, this has led me to be a recognizable face in my local grocery stores and a chronic impulse buyer/overspender*), and so that we could afford a house with central air conditioning—I was so tired of the Georgia heat! I also desperately wanted a car so I could go wherever I wanted, *whenever I wanted* and *never, ever* have to wait for anyone to pick me up or have to leave a place early because someone else was ready to go. Finally, I *never, ever* wanted to see the look that I saw on some people's faces when I told them where I lived… Underwood Homes—also known as *"The Bottom."*

I am not joking, this is literally how people referred to the neighborhood where I spent most of my childhood, and it is a neighborhood that was so drug/crime-ridden that until recently, my mother and I were even afraid for me to drive through it… Now that there are plans to tear it down, my mother and I finally drove through it with my sons. It looked worse than I remembered, but it brought back a lot of memories… Unfortunately, most of those memories were of me being sad, lonely, angry, and frustrated, especially where my weight was concerned. In hindsight, I think a number of the issues that I have had to deal with and work through over the years during my journey toward "happiness" originated from this time in my life…

Ghosts from My Past

My parents separated when I was four and divorced when I was seven. My father, God rest his soul, *died in 2006*. He was an alcoholic, who physically abused my mother, and after the divorce he never played a role in my life— *physically, emotionally, or financially*. I **never** saw or heard from him on my birthday, Thanksgiving, or Christmas. There were no calls, cards, or gifts either. He never attended plays, band performances or awards programs. He wasn't at my high school or college graduations (*he didn't even know what college I went to until someone told him*) or my wedding, and although it hurt, I was somewhat glad because his drinking, bad behavior, and run-ins with the law were always a *huge* source of embarrassment for me.

Be that as it may, *I still recall longing to see him even though he lived less than ten miles from us…* The pain caused by this longing was made even worse by one seemingly harmless question—*When was the last time you saw your ole' daddy?* I don't know if people realized how much rage and sadness was generated over the years from this one question about my father. If they did, I don't think they would have asked a seven-year-old or even a fourteen-year-old this question. *Didn't anyone ever see the look on my face?* I thought someone might understand the pain and embarrassment a child would suffer from answering *"I don't know"* repeatedly over the years, especially when it may have been asked in front of other children who had fathers in their lives. Every child wants to be loved or at least acknowledged by his or her father, and if that can't happen, maybe the child should be able to at least mourn or deal with that fact in private, *not with the world watching…*

It didn't seem that anyone had a clue or even cared. To make matters worse, some would laugh as they asked *the question* yet again. When I would try to change the subject, they would go into a story of what he was doing the last time they saw him (e.g., he was drunk, he was riding a bike instead of driving a car, he was beaten up, he was in jail, etc.). *Why?* This one question constantly opened *the wound that never healed.* In fact, each time I was asked, it felt like someone had poked me with a hot branding iron. The truly sad part is that I heard it asked over and over during my childhood and teenage years... The pain from it made me almost hate the askers of the question, and I think this could be one of the reasons why I never developed deep connections or relationships with many of the people in my family... This was certainly an eye-opener, as I had often wondered what happened to those relationships—*why was/am I so detached from almost all of them?* I didn't understand those feelings then, *but I do now...*

Metaphorically, I think the branding iron reference is very appropriate and significant because each time someone asked me *the question*, a piece of my self-esteem was chipped away. It was as if I were being branded *The Child of a Loser and destined to turn out the same way*. I never even knew until I had children of my own how much it hurt me *and still hurts* on some levels... However, it is obvious as I struggle to watch movies such as *Father of the Bride* with Steve Martin or listen to Luther Vandross' *Dance with My Father*. This hurt is also at the heart of my strong warning to my children regarding friends or relatives where they have never met a child's father or have never heard a child speak of his or her father: *If a child wants to discuss his or her father, let the child do it, not you...* They know I am serious too. *I find it interesting that the kids that I was thinking of have never mentioned their fathers.* They seem to operate as if their fathers don't exist, which is how I would have preferred it, and it is how I operated for much of my life.

It has been very hard for me to get to the point where I am today, where I don't hate my father, and I actually have some level of forgiveness/understanding/compassion toward him. However, I have often found myself burdened with a lot of emotional baggage resulting from *his choice* not to be a part of my life. Because I never used to acknowledge or talk about this *baggage*, I believe the hurt festered below the surface for many years without my realizing it, but it manifested itself in many subtle ways... This was probably the source of much of my anger, isolation and rebellion during my teen years. As a result, I wound up spending a lot of time alone and eating a lot, but never understanding why. I realize now that I was looking for acceptance and love on so many different levels... *from my father, my mother, relatives, and friends*, but I could never seem to find it. I think this may be why there have not been a lot of people I have been close to or felt comfortable with over the years.

Growing up as an only child (*my father had two other children while he was married to my mother, but I only met them once or twice*) in a very "loose-knit" family only added to my feelings of isolation. My father was also an only child, so there were no aunts and uncles or close cousins my age on his side of the family. However, he did have first cousins, whose kids I wound up spending time with during my late teens. My mother had a larger family, but they were a different story altogether. She had eight brothers and sisters, but my grandmother (*God rest her soul*) raised them in such a way that no one seemed comfortable showing any real affection to each other. To my knowledge there has never been a family reunion among the group, and I can't recall many happy memories with them. When I was with them as a child, I always felt *less than* because of the way they talked about my father in front of me. These feelings, coupled with the fact that I never told anyone that I was sexually molested by a family "friend" (*if you can call him that*) when I was nine, only made me drift even further. In this day and age, a child with similar problems might be in therapy. However, my issues went unnoticed because I didn't "*act out*," everything was internalized. I didn't have behavioral problems or anything like that, and I was a pretty good kid aside from the fact that I was noticeably angry with almost everyone in my family. I also had a sarcastic tone and a smart mouth when talking to most of the adults in my family, especially my mother. *OK, so maybe I did act out a little.*

The Weight of *Who I Was*

Thinking back to this period, I do not remember telling anyone about my inner turmoil because very few adults ever asked what was going on with me or seemed interested in my life, and if they weren't interested enough to ask, I didn't bother to tell them—*anything.* Also, because my mother worked a lot, and we were both too strong-willed to meet each other in the middle on areas where we disagreed, there was almost zero communication between us regarding anything that might have been bothering me. I also didn't have friends that I felt comfortable enough with to talk about serious topics, so I kept everything that hurt to myself.

I think this is one of the reasons that up until the time I met my husband, I was a loner. I think it may have been because I felt like no one really cared about me. I know now that people did, but back then I couldn't see or feel it, and my actions and attitudes reflected that belief. Believing that no one cares about you feels almost as if there is a hole in your soul, and the sweetness, innocence, and trust of a child starts to seep out… A lot of the niceness and loving-kindness I had as a child went away, and the girl that was left in her place was quick to anger, argumentative, critical, contrary, defensive, guarded, and *full of issues*.

As people with internalized issues tend to do, I found an escape—fortunately it was books and reading. Reading has always been a wonderful way for me to mentally run away from whatever is bothering me. So the Augusta Library became my second home, and some of the best memories from my youth are the hours I spent there *alone* reading. That sounds sad even to my own ears, but it's true, especially during my early teens… The library was a place to hide and dream. It also served as a life preserver for my dreams, as well as laid the groundwork for me to be a good student and later go on to and finish college. However, aside from academics, not a whole lot else was going on in my life then…

Even though I was a pretty fast runner, I never ran track or participated in sports. I never told anyone the reason back then, but it was because you needed a ride to/from practice and sporting events, *and* we didn't have a car. You also needed money for uniforms and other incidentals, which we just didn't have. Because I didn't feel like taking on the stress of all of these seemingly impossible obstacles, I did nothing unless it was cheap or free, **and** I could see a definite way to get a ride to/from the events. These restrictions led me to play the flute in the band. *Why the band?* Because my mother got the band instructor to agree to bring me home after practice (this was appreciated, but was another source of embarrassment). *Why the flute?* Because you didn't have to buy any extra equipment (e.g., reeds, mouthpiece, etc.). *Cheap and free, that's how it had to be.* Today as I look at the money and time my husband and I devote to sports and activities for our boys, I realize that they cannot ever comprehend or relate to my experiences, but then again, *I never wanted them to…*

I know it may be hard to believe, but the frustration and worry caused by not having a car of our own was one of the major stressors of my childhood and teen years. Almost every school event or activity (e.g., band performances, award ceremonies, pep rallies, football games, dances, etc.) had me scrambling to figure out how I was going to get where I needed or wanted to be **and** then to get back home. Trying to figure this all out on my own (*my mom does not drive, and we could not afford a car, my dad was not around, and no relatives lived close enough where I could ask for help*) caused me a great a deal of stress because as any other teenager, I wanted to go places, do exciting things and have fun. However, if the destination wasn't on a bus line and being held during the day, I simply could not go. This limitation caused me to miss a lot of school functions that I actually looked forward to.

One of those events was Superlatives Night during my senior year in high school when I was nominated for the *Most Likely to Succeed*, *Most Studious* and *Most Ladyl*ike awards. My closest friend at the time, who lived in my neighborhood and was also nominated for these awards, went, but because she didn't offer me a ride, I was too proud to ask her or her family for a ride. It felt too much like begging, and after feeling that way a lot during my childhood with my uncles, my grandmother and *her*, I was too proud to beg by this point… *So because I was too proud to ask*, I missed it.

I won at least two out of the three awards, but I had to pick them up from school afterwards. As usual, I made up some excuse about being busy that night. You may think I am being melodramatic, but incidents like this seriously marred my teenage experience because to live in places like Augusta, Georgia you *really* need a car. This is why I only went to *one* football game during high school, and even that outing had its problems: my great-uncle dropped me off, and I resorted to taking a ride from a stranger to get back home. He could have been Ted Bundy for all I knew, but I got in the car with him because I didn't feel like I had any alternatives that wouldn't hurt my pride. Having to go to such lengths just to go somewhere socially was just too much to worry about, and sitting somewhere hoping to get a ride home is no fun whatsoever. In fact, it was very stressful *and embarrassing*, especially when asking for a ride home meant telling people where I lived and seeing some hesitate as they pondered the prospect of going to my neighborhood. So after a while, I just pretended I wasn't interested in going to school activities and wound up spending many weekends sitting home alone watching T.V., reading and eating, *usually all three* for most of my middle and high school years.

Fortunately, a program called *Upward Bound*, designed for economically disadvantaged students, helped me to temporarily break this cycle. It was held on the campus of Paine College in Augusta, Georgia (*the first college I had ever seen in person*), and it opened a whole new world of possibility for me. I sat in on college classes, and there were refresher courses/tutoring during the summer and the school year to help prepare us for college. There were trips (e.g., my first time going to the skating rink, the World's Fair and to Florida theme parks), activities, and *freedom*. Believe it or not, these were all life-changing opportunities that helped me to escape and *forget for a time…*

The Young Woman *I Became*

People who knew me then, and who know me now, have no idea of the stress, worry and hurt I hid. Over time, it turned into anger and rage bubbling below the surface… I think this can easily happen to children who grow up feeling that no one cares about them—*negative feelings/energy just keep building inside*. This is what I think happens to many inner-city youth who do not have a positive outlet for these types of feelings. Although I cannot condone hurting others because you are hurting, I can really relate to some of these young people who are obviously hurting, but have no positive outlet to express it. In too many cases, if nothing changes in the situation, the negative feelings wind up being directed at the closest target… For this reason I am so thankful that I have always had a strong desire to achieve/excel; otherwise, I could have gone down a very wrong and different path… In fact, as I look back, I can certainly understand why my mind has blanked out some of the details from my past.

Isn't it amazing how so many little episodes from the past can shape who we are without us even realizing it? We are truly the sum of our experiences—*whether we realize it or not*. Some of the ways we have been shaped may be obvious, while others are not as obvious… For example, how could a Black girl living in the projects wind up with a voice like Mr. Bill (*the cookie character from Saturday Night Live during the days of Eddie Murphy and Dan Aykroyd, famous for saying "Oooh Nooo"*)? How is it that this same girl sat in the house alone *excitedly* watching *Little House on the Prairie*, *The Waltons*, *Andy Griffith*, *Gilligan's Island*, *What's Happening* and *Good Times*, while listening to not only Diana Ross and Luther Vandross, but also Barbara Streisand, Barry Manilow, and *Neil Diamond*? I can't even recall what led me to have such eclectic tastes. *I've just always been weird.*

However, as an adult, I realize that the weirdness that separated me was actually a blessing because anyone on the wrong path usually would never even think to include me or let me know what they were up to. Not saying that I have never done stupid things as a kid, *because I certainly have*, but for the most part, no matter how troubled I may have been, I have never wanted to be *in trouble*. I have always wanted to excel and be successful at *SOMETHING*. I didn't always know exactly *what* I wanted to be successful at or how I would achieve it... But, I can tell you that these little quirks, coupled with the fact that I could not go out of the house *and* no one could come in until my mother came home from work, *shaped* me into a less-than-popular teenager. This was the point when experiences from the past began to shape my future:

Emotional Issues + Unpopular Teenager = Stay-In-The-House-And-Eat-Nonstop

This was a formula for disaster. My weight started to creep... Stretch marks began to appear in noticeable places such as the backs of my calves... I was so embarrassed. By the time I went to high school I was in the 150s. At five foot seven, this weight might not have been so bad if I had lots of curves to balance it out, but I didn't. **This was *the* absolute worst period of my life, and I had no idea how to change any of it.** I didn't feel good about my weight, my hair, my clothes, my family, where I lived, or my life in general... The only thing I felt good about was my mind and the academic achievement I experienced. So without any answers or options that worked, I continued doing what I was doing: *sitting in the house alone, watching TV, reading, and* **eating nonstop**. This pattern continued for years until a series of interesting life events revealed a path to help me become the slim person I was in my daydreams.

These *revelations* happened in stages over the course of fifteen years, and I like to think of them as *wake-up calls*. So far, I have had three major wake-up calls with my weight over the years that have made me look in the mirror in desperation and say, "*I don't wanna go out like this!*" These *wake-up calls*, or whatever you want to call them, helped me to formulate a plan that changed the way I feel about myself, how I eat, and how active I am, which enables me to keep my weight within a reasonable/healthy range to this day. What I learned and am about to share may not be the most profound thing you have ever heard, but it has been *life-changing* for me nonetheless, and I believe it can be for you as well…

~

Chapter 3

R e f l e c t   &   R e d i s c o v e r
(S t e p   1)

Now that you have a better idea of who I am, I thought it might be helpful for you to know the wake-up calls or points of inspiration that motivated me to look in the mirror and say, ***"The person at this weight is not who I am—I have to do something different."*** I can remember having this realization at three distinct times in my life:

- Wake-Up Call #1 / *The Young & Pudgy Phase*
- Wake-Up Call #2 / *The Baby-Weight Battle*
- Wake-Up Call #3 / *The Spinning Out of Control Phase*

I think these stories will help you in your own life as you see *how* I came to be overweight in three different circumstances and how I fought back and won—*without diets, paying for expensive food plans, or living at the gym.* The purpose of this chapter is to show you that *you can lose the weight, no matter what the circumstances.* I share a lot of details because I don't want to gloss over the struggle or make it seem like it was easy, *because it wasn't.* It was a fight, and sometimes it still is, but it has been well worth it. *I know it will be for you as well.*

This is why step one of my *Healthy Weight for Life®* program is for you to *Reflect & Rediscover…* You must *reflect* over your life experiences so you can understand how you wound up where you are with your weight today... *What led you here? Why are you eating the way you are? Are you the person you thought you'd be?* Well if you aren't, don't you think it's time to re*discover* the person you wanted to be? The happy, purpose-filled, successful person you are/were in your dreams. Well this is the chapter where you start the inner work that is required to get you started on the path to becoming that person where your weight is concerned.

I wish the process were easier, but you have to know "who you are" right at this moment in order for you to become who and what you want to be in the future... ***This is a critical step, so please don't skip it.*** In the meantime, I hope my stories and examples entertain and encourage you, as well as help to inspire your self-reflection and rediscovery efforts. So let's get on with the story and get you on your way.

~❧~

Wake-Up Call #1
The Young & Pudgy Phase
~ · ~ · ~ ~ · ~ · ~ · ~

I had just finished my first year at Clemson University, which I felt was a major accomplishment for a kid coming from the projects without significant financial/emotional support from my family. However, a lot of stress came along with that accomplishment—being in a strange place on my own, feeling a little uneasy in an environment where there were very few Black faces, and with the slow realization that I had chosen the wrong major. I was definitely out of my element, unlike the students I saw who seemed more prepared in every way. Many of them experienced comforts and lifestyles I had only seen on television—*cars, expenses paid before they got there, families they could call for money/help,* and *parents, grandparents, and siblings who came to visit and tailgate during games.* My life was so far removed from this—I couldn't even begin to relate.

As I took all of this in some of my family members were telling my mother she should "*make*" me come home and get a job because we could not afford college. This was ridiculous—**they weren't paying for it, I was**! So no one was going to make me do anything I didn't want to do. In fact, I decided that I was *never* going to let them, or anyone else, put me down again or dissuade me from pursuing my dreams. *Not without a fight!* Well, years of fighting with my family left me *very* angry and bitter toward all of them. I don't know about other families, but I was amazed at how critical/unsupportive my relatives were before and during college. I remember wishing that they might pull together to help me at some point… I could never quite wrap my mind around the fact that they could point out our inability to pay for college, but never offer to help… I never asked anyone why. *Also, I rarely mentioned, thought of, or went home…*

However, as I watched friends and relatives my age who had parents helping them go to college, as well as boyfriends and close friends around them, I will admit I was very envious—of their money (*no matter how little it might have been*), their friends and boyfriends, as well as the peace of mind that comes from knowing someone at home has your back and is there to help you if you need it. I always wanted that peace of mind, and I have to admit that I was tired of always feeling alone and having to handle everything on my own. Also, looking back at this period, I realize that there has always been something in my personality that makes it difficult for me to form lasting, close friendships, so my first few years of college were very lonely.

Combine all of this with the uncertainty of whether I would have enough money for tuition and expenses after piecing together scholarships, grants, loans, and money from summer jobs, it was a pretty scary time for me. I was usually faced at least once a semester with the warning, "*You need $X thousands by Friday, or you will be sent home.*" Each time this happened, I would leave the Financial Aid Office, take my last few dollars (*I had very little left after paying for books and essential items*) and go to *The Clemson House*, which sold the best cheeseburgers and tater tots for only $5.25. I would take the food back to my room and eat it while I watched *All My Children*. After I ate, I'd say a quick prayer to ask God for help, and then I would go to sleep. As soon as I woke up, I would head back to the Financial Aid Office, and each time, *somehow, some way*, with God's help, the financial problems were always resolved. I was completely amazed each time this happened because most times I even wound up with extra money for clothes, spending money to last *almost* until I got my income tax refund, *and* even some to send home! I think this is how the phrase "*Praise the Lord*" became, and still is today, a regular part of my everyday language because for me to go from "*not enough*" to "*more than enough*" each year was nothing short of a miracle.

Stress & More Stress

Even though most of my financial problems were usually resolved, the constant financial rollercoaster as well as other factors caused me a tremendous

amount of stress. One of the most pressing factors was my choice of majors…
For three years I studied electrical engineering when I really wanted, and was
more suited academically, to study journalism. However, I picked my major
based on the highest starting salary I could find because, quite honestly, I
was tired of being poor. So my major was not chosen based on my interests,
passion, or academic strengths; it was determined by economics and my desire
to get an engineering summer internship with E.I. DuPont (*a job that helped
pay for my books and basic necessities during my first two years of college and gave me
valuable job experience on my resume after college*). Needless to say, I struggled
academically. I did very well in English, literature, and public speaking classes,
but calculus, physics, and engineering classes such as statics and dynamics (the
study of vectors, *I think*)—you could forget about it! I wasn't fooling anyone,
but I continued on hoping things would improve. I had only two options—
continue on and get my degree or give up, and go back to Augusta in defeat
and hear family say, "*We told you so.*" There was no way I would **ever** let that
happen! It was all or nothing. **Going back home empty-handed was not
an option!**

Unintentional Deception

As I continued on with my all-or-nothing attitude, I may have seemed fine
on the outside, but I had a lot of inner struggles going on regarding my financial
situation, my family, my grades, and the shame I felt whenever I went back to
the projects and my old way of life. While I was in school, for the most part, no
one knew where or how I lived, no one knew about my father… People just saw
me as I was there and made their own assumptions. I never lied, but I never gave
more information than was asked of me. So I guess I kind of lived a double life,
as most assumed that I could actually afford to be there and that I had money
because I wore nice clothes *and* often had more spending money than some of
them. *They didn't know the money was left over from grants, scholarships, and loans once
they all finally came in.* People tend to make assumptions about my background,
then and now, because of the way I talk, act, and dress—many have assumed that I
grew up with money and had a pretty easy life. When *asked*, I was always honest,
but most people thought I was joking. It was actually funny after a while because
no one really believed me when I told them I was poor, no matter how hard I
tried to convince them.

As this continued, I think I started to experience some sort of temporary psychosis where I almost brainwashed myself into forgetting what my real story was. *I actually liked their version better anyway.* During those first few years I felt like a different person when I was at school, like I had finally escaped my *less-than-impressive* past. However, when I went home and found myself riding the bus in Augusta again (*you only ride the bus there if you don't drive or can't afford a car*) or helping my mother clean the homes of suburban White families, some of whom had children, relatives, or friends who went to Clemson, *my real life was right there waiting for me.* I know you can't escape your past, but I see now I was definitely trying...

Alright, I know what you are thinking... I shouldn't have been embarrassed, but when you are young, **you can allow** your peers to make you feel inferior, and there were times when *I allowed* that to happen. In fact, I remember when a suburban friend's family gave me a ride back to school one semester. They came to my house because I couldn't get a ride to theirs. I will never forget how my friend looked when she saw where I lived. She looked almost as if I had been deceitful because I never looked/sounded/acted as if I came from the projects. She seemed surprised, and after the shock wore off, she seemed almost amused. Of course she had jokes and comments, even if they were subtle. I was embarrassed beyond words, and it felt like her perception of me had changed. It could have been in my mind, but *it didn't feel that way.*

That turned out to be a fateful ride back to school because other people found out shortly thereafter and began to talk, which only added to my increasing stress and isolation. I don't know why it matters either way, but I have noticed that some people treat you differently when they find out you have less than they do... One of my relationships with a cousin was actually damaged beyond repair because someone she knew at Clemson told her that I was there pretending that I was rich when really I wasn't. I never pretended anything, but I didn't let my background define me, *and* I was too embarrassed to tell my whole story... Unbelievably some people seemed even angry as the information circulated over the years, and if they were mad at me, they might say things like, "*She thinks she is so much, but she ain't nobody, knowing her [butt] comes from the project!*" Ouch, that hurt!

Exposed and Headed for Trouble

Things really started to unravel toward the end of my sophomore year… This was the semester when I shared a room with a girl who was in love with a star basketball player (he later went on to play in the NBA). To me, it *seemed* like they were *always* in our room, and *three was definitely a crowd…* As a result, I spent a lot of time sitting in the lobby of our building watching TV, and studying. This made me really sad because it felt like I was sitting on the sidelines watching as everyone else enjoyed their college experience, doing all the things I saw people do in TV show portrayals of college life (e.g., partying, dating, pledging sororities, going to pep rallies, etc.). All of the things I dreamt I'd be doing in college, *but wasn't.*

Unfortunately my new hangout was one floor away from a fully stocked vending machine. I have to tell you, *this was not the best place for a displaced, stressed, and lonely girl to be…* When I lived at home we could not afford to buy Twinkies, Ho-Hos, doughnuts, and two or three types of chips on a regular basis, so when I saw this machine, it was as if a bright light from heaven shone on it, and angels started singing a chorus of "Hallelujah." I LITERALLY LOST MY MIND! I did not know how to act with sweet temptation being that close. I was so bored and lonely, and I really wished I could find someone like my roommate did. *Poor me! Why didn't I have a boyfriend? Why was I always alone? Why was I stuck in this doggone lobby???*

This line of thinking made me feel sorry for myself, which made me want to eat even more. So every time I found myself stuck in that lobby, I would also *find* myself "visiting" the machine just to see what new treat might have been added, and the next thing you know, I was showing ALL THE WAY out! I would even "visit" the machine when no one was in my room, and with each *visit* I would buy something. What's worse, I would also usually buy a soda as well. Pretty soon I was acting as if the vending machine was my *friend*. What sense does that make? *Absolutely none!* As a result, I walked away with a very valuable lesson that I carry with me to this day: **vending machines are not our friends**, especially if we have any kind of weight problem. Most of us do not need to buy snacks from machines on a daily basis (e.g., chips, cookies, candy bars, sodas, etc.)—doing so can definitely lead to more trouble. I did try to get a handle on the situation by forcing myself to walk up the ten flights of stairs to my room after some of my *visits,* but that still didn't stop me. I was trying to fill a void in my life with vending machine snacks, and although it wasn't working, *I kept right on eating…*

After a few months of this craziness, I went home with my 11/12 clothes so tight I could barely breathe. I remember the embarrassment I felt as relatives and friends commented on my weight, especially when my neighbor (a lady who weighed almost two hundred pounds) looked at me, and said, "*What, are you trying to get fat?*" I got on the scale, and my *secret* actions definitely had *very public* consequences—I had gone from the 150s to the 160s since my last visit home! That was my first real wake-up call, and it forced me to take a long, hard look in the mirror and realize that I needed to get it together. Carrying that much weight around was very uncomfortable, and the person I had become was not who I wanted to be. I knew I needed to leave the vending machines alone, and I needed to exercise, but more importantly, I needed to do something to minimize stress and to deal with my feelings of loneliness and displacement.

To get the ball rolling, I started looking for people to spend time with and activities other than watching TV when my room was off-limits. If I was lonely or sad, I started walking to a drug store that was about a mile away to buy whatever magazine I could afford. I am, and have always been, a sucker for magazines. This new routine of weaning myself from the vending machine and walking more frequently got me back to 152 pounds, which I was thankful for, but my continual prayer was still that one day I would wake up miraculously 15 pounds lighter, and be in the 130s… You may think I am joking, but I actually asked the Lord to do this for me because I have never had enough willpower to diet. *What can I say, I was desperate.*

Time for a Change…

While I waited for the miracle weight loss thing to happen, I continued on with my life while soul-searching on what I wanted for the future. I started to accept the fact that electrical engineering was not for me, and the first few thoughts of an exit strategy from that major began to take shape. I think my "magazine walks" not only helped me manage stress better and get back into the

150s, but they also helped me to get in touch with my true feelings regarding what I wanted for my life. As a result, at the start of my junior year, I looked into transferring to the University of South Carolina (USC) to study journalism, as writing and talking are my real passions. I even entertained the idea of becoming a news anchor or some other type of broadcast journalist. However, after getting my butt royally kicked by the engineering classes, I didn't have the 3.0 GPA needed to make the switch (*this fact also ended my internship with DuPont*). The switch might not have been such a good idea anyway because it would have been a form of curricular-suicide, as my math and science foundation was not as impressive in the journalism realm. I would have basically been starting over, which was not an option, as my Georgia-Pacific scholarship was only for four years.

If I am being completely honest here, another reason I considered transferring to USC was because it had three times Clemson's student population, and I thought it would improve the odds of me finding my future husband. After all, my cousin was dating her future husband, who was an engineering student there. She also went there for weekend visits, and it seemed like she was having such a great time. Maybe it was the place for me too... I just had such a strong belief (*borderline obsession*) that college was where you met your future husband. *Isn't that what happened in those happily-ever-after movies from the '60s?* So for the first time ever, I am admitting to the world that I went to college looking for a bachelor of science (BS) ***and*** an *MRS* degree. I wanted it all—a degree that would lead me to a high-paying job and a husband that would lead me to the family I always wanted. There I said it! My husband knew after the fact, but this was definitely not information I shared with a lot of people...

Because fate/grades prevented me from transferring and drastically changing my major, I decided to stay at Clemson and finish what I started. However, I knew I would never get out of there with a degree in electrical engineering, so I started looking for majors that required the same foundational background as an engineering degree. This led me to a relatively new major at the time, computer information systems, which allowed all of the calculus, chemistry, and physics I had taken to count. This also seemed to make sense because although DuPont required me to major in an engineering discipline, all of my jobs were in the area of computer science. I liked this major because it didn't have as many computer classes, which was good because I never was a *"sold-out"* computer science student/professional. I only had a minor interest, and there were only so many courses I could get in before graduation. So this was definitely the best path to take, and I believe the Lord threw me a number of life preservers to help me continue on.

Help from an Unlikely Source

One of those *life preservers* came to me in the form of an unknowing angel… During one of my summer school experiences, I found myself short as usual. It was for the monumental sum of $360. Regardless of the amount, I went through all of my usual steps with the Financial Aid Office. *Of course they already knew me there as often as I had been there for help in the past.* I even had a work-study job there, and one of the employees was the matron of honor at my wedding! So when I tell you I exhausted every means possible in terms of financial aid, *you'd better believe it!* Once we had pursued all options they could think of (e.g., deferments, grants, emergency student loans, etc.), they told me to go talk to my counselor. I think this was a nice way of saying, *"Please go away and bother someone else! We have told you a hundred different ways that we can't help you!"*

At that point, I had to listen because even I couldn't think of anything else they could do to help. So I took their advice and went to bug/talk to my counselor. I had never talked to him other than to ask him to sign off on my schedule, but that day I was prepared to bug him until he helped me come up with another solution. So I stood outside of his office waiting for him to return, and after about an hour of waiting patiently, another professor came out of his office to ask if there was anything he could do. I told him that I was waiting for my counselor, but thanks anyway. After I waited a little bit longer, he came back and asked if I was sure there was nothing he could do until my counselor was back in the office. After he asked a second time and invited me into his office, I finally unloaded all of my troubles on him as well as all of the things I had done thus far to find a solution. As you already know from reading this book, *I give a lot of details*, and my story to him was no different. However, he got to see my face and hear the desperation of someone determined not to be sent home.

After I had talked for at least twenty minutes straight, he looked at me and said, "It certainly sounds like you have pursued every possible option… *Isn't there anyone from home you could call? Your father? Anyone else from your family?* I abruptly answered, "*No, there is no one else.*" This seemed to intrigue him, as he asked me yet again, "*There is no one in your family that can or will help you?*" Again, I said no because people might have given me the occasional gifts of money for graduation, but there was no one I knew that had ever offered to give/loan me money for school. In fact, the one time my mother arranged for an uncle to help with a $200 loan, he was asking her (*in front of people*) when I was going to pay it back within a few months. I was angry, but I agreed to repay him with interest when I got my tax refund. Once I got it, he happily accepted the principal *and interest* for the loan. At that point I vowed I would never look to him or any other family member for help. *No one offered, so I never asked…* So when the professor asked again, I blankly reiterated, "*That is not an option.*"

After I answered all of his questions in the greatest of detail, he pulled his chair back from his desk and said, "Well, I have a symposium (*this was the first time I had ever heard that word*) to go to…" Immediately I thought, "*Why on earth did I waste my time on this man?*" Still I stood up, shook his hand, and I thanked him for listening. I also said something like I hoped he enjoyed his symposium, and I immediately started thinking of what I was going to do next. It really was a do-or-die situation for me because if I didn't take that computer science class, I would definitely not graduate in the five-year timeline my new major committed me to. My thoughts were racing so much that I didn't even realize that he had pulled out his checkbook…

He started writing, and then he handed me a check for half of the amount I owed. I was in total shock! However, as I started excitedly thanking him, I shamefully remember thinking, "*This is great, but how am I going to get the other half?*" As if he read my mind, he started writing a second check for the other half! He explained that the first half was a scholarship that he was giving me because he thought it would be a shame for someone like me to be sent home. He said it was obvious that I was very intelligent and had a lot of potential. He also said he was impressed by how logical my thought process was as I explained *all* of the paths I had pursued to solve my problem. I have to tell you, as a *Black* girl from the projects of Augusta, Georgia, I was astounded by the fact that a *White* professor, whom I had never met, would give me money for school when my own family wouldn't. Based on my upbringing and experiences, I don't know what I expected from him, but I certainly wasn't expecting this!

As he gave me the second check, he explained that it was a loan that I could repay one year from that date. *However, unlike my uncle he would not accept any interest.* I was amazed, and I have to admit that I did wonder *why* he would do something like this for me. In fact, I was downright suspicious, especially when he told me there were a couple of conditions. *Uh oh, here it comes, I thought...* I should have known it was too good to be true! In order to get the money, I had to agree not to tell anyone what he had done for me because no one would believe that he did it just out of the kindness of his heart. I could definitely understand that because even I was suspicious. As hard as it was, I never told anyone at Clemson, or at home, what he did for me, *and* I did repay him at the end of one year. The other condition I had to honor was that in the future I would help another underprivileged student the same way. Although my husband and I have done this for some people on their way to/through college, I still plan to contact Clemson's Financial Aid Office to formally set something up to do just that. It is something I must do because his assistance meant the world to me, and I would love to help someone else in the same way. I don't know if the professor knew it or not, but his vote of confidence, in the form of money, did wonders for my self-esteem.

Full Steam Ahead

Once everything was *somewhat* on track for me to get a degree in a high-paying industry, the task of obtaining my other degree (an *MRS*) required my attention. I could not leave Clemson without knowing who my future husband would be. Not only did I want financial success, I also wanted a family, and for me, that starts with a husband. So the search for my future husband officially began. Being the compulsive person that I am, I made a list, which wound up being the equivalent of a letter/prayer to God. In my letter, I told Him what I was looking for in my future husband *in great detail*. It started off as a short list, but I am sure, as you can imagine, it quickly turned into almost five pages! *My future husband would be honest, loyal, trustworthy, and affectionate... He would like to hold hands… He would like to laugh. He would be my friend. He would be attractive to me (color/ethnicity did not matter). He would like to go to church (even though I was a heathen at the time). He would be my height in heels, his calves had to be my size or larger (I have very muscular calves, and I just could not see myself with a man whose calves were smaller than mine).* The list went on and on, but I was very specific about the qualities I wanted in my life mate and the father of my children.

The list/prayer, whatever you want to call it, even covered areas I wanted to change about myself… *I was going to lose the glasses and get contacts. I was going to change my style of dress to be younger and more alluring* (translation miniskirts with high heels). I have to admit I wore very conservative clothes that were more appropriate for work/my internships (e.g., long skirts, moderate heels, etc.). *I was going to change my hair too, and at some point I would find a way to get it healthier and grow it longer. I also planned to be more carefree and adventurous*—even if I didn't have friends to go to parties with, I would go alone if I had to, but I was determined to be out there and open to meet my future husband.

You can laugh if you want to because I do realize that I am crazy, compulsive, and little fanatical once I set my mind on something, and my mind was set on finding a husband! I knew no other way to get what I wanted other than to give it 100 percent. My dreams were fueled by all of the Harlequin Romance books I read during the summers of my teenage years. I am embarrassed now to even admit that I read, *still read*, Harlequin Romance books from time to time, mainly on the treadmill. What can I say? I have always been a sucker for happy endings. That is still true today—whether it is movies or books. I am always looking for a happy ending, and that is what I have always wanted for my life as well. This naïve optimism is what had me thinking that my Prince Charming was just out there waiting for me to find him!

<u>Prince Charming?</u>

During the fall semester, I finally got a chance to try out my new look and confidence at one of the fraternity parties on campus. Even though I did not have any friends who wanted to go with me, I decided that I would go anyway, *by myself!* Even though I was alone, I felt in my element. I think it was because, for the first time, I really liked the way I looked *even though I had not lost any weight.*

31

Somehow I had started to feel more comfortable in my own skin. This was the first party I ever even considered going to alone much less actually going there by myself. However, I wasn't nervous. For the first time I felt really alive and *vivacious. When and how* did that happen? Not sure, but my hair was teased high (*think Oprah in the '80s*), my skirt was short, my sweater was fitted, my heels were high and my eyes and lips were highlighted by my makeup and lack of glasses. I walked around talking to people I knew and *asking guys to dance* when my favorite songs came on. I was feeling pretty good about myself, and I remember thinking this new independence/confidence thing felt good, and then BAM!

I literally turned around, and I saw the most beautiful hazel green eyes I had ever seen! Then before I knew what I was saying, I said, "*WOW, you have the most beautiful eyes I have ever seen! Would you like to dance?*" He was the cutest, sweetest guy I had ever met. He liked me. I liked him, and after a few weeks *I* was in love! *I* wanted to marry him and have his children *even though he didn't even remember my last name!* Nevertheless, we became best friends, and eventually my best friend became my boyfriend (*I'll tell you that story later*)! More importantly, *he liked me for who I was, and* he thought I was beautiful! I couldn't believe it! My dream guy actually thought I was beautiful, *and* he LOVED me! I didn't have to change or try to impress him. He accepted me for me... What an unimaginable and unexpected blessing! Also, isn't it an interesting coincidence that this type of relationship never happened for me until I accepted myself as I was? I *think this is a valuable lesson for anyone who is looking for a relationship.*

The Final Frontier

Finally I was on the right path to an MRS degree as well as a BS degree! *Now if only I could just lose the fifteen pounds that didn't seem to bother my boyfriend, but were driving me crazy!* Why are we never happy? You accomplish one goal, and then immediately your mind moves onto something else. I was happier than I had ever been in my entire life, but I still desperately wanted to lose weight. I just didn't know how. For a time I just sat around fantasizing about a magic pill or a miracle from God that would take the weight off for me practically overnight. However, I didn't want to do the work required to lose the weight and keep it off (i.e., change my eating habits and exercise).

To come to my defense, even though I was misguided *and lazy*, I did realize that it was foolishness to think that God would just *cause* me to lose fifteen pounds without me changing my eating habits and exercising consistently. Nevertheless, this didn't keep me from bugging Him about it anyway. In the meantime, I continued eating any and every snack, treat, or fast-food item I wanted*, whenever I wanted*. However, after a while I noticed that when I ate my usual eight-pack of strawberry cream cookies with a sixteen-ounce *Coke* as an afternoon snack, I felt yuck, almost queasy. It seems that after a while "*something*" said to me, "*Do you really need to drink a large soda with those cookies?*" Believe it or not, I actually spent time pondering the question, and I realized that it was ridiculously greedy, especially for someone who *claimed* she wanted to lose weight! As a result, since I would never give up my eight-pack of cookies, I felt compelled to try drinking water with them instead, and you know what? *It was really good!*

This was a major revelation for me, as I did not grow up in an environment where people just sat around drinking water. If you were drinking water that meant you did not have *ANYTHING* else—you were all out of *Kool-Aid*, ice tea, soda, lemonade, *and* juice. *Water was always the last resort.* However, after this experience a lifelong habit was formed where I have a large glass of ice water whenever I eat something sweet. Also, because I was such a sweets addict, I wound up drinking a whole lot of ice water and liking it. Guess what else? After I stopped having sweets with soda, I noticed that the queasy feeling I used to get went away. As a result, water became my favorite drink, soda took a well-deserved backseat, and I never felt better! This has been one of the most life-changing decisions I have ever made. I am so glad I learned this lesson early because now my sons also drink more water than any other drink—at first it was by force, but it has become the drink they reach for most. *Don't think I am saying my sons wouldn't drink soda nonstop if I let them, but at least they don't mind drinking water.*

Other Changes to Come
As I got used to the "water" thing, I felt compelled to look at other areas of my daily diet that I could improve while still eating what I wanted. In fact, one day while grocery shopping, I saw sandwich breads that had half the calories of

regular bread for the first time. It seems that *"something"* said to me, *"You eat a lot of sandwiches, why not try switching to the low-calorie bread?"* It was only a few cents more, so I thought, *"Why not?"* Surprisingly, it tasted the same, and next thing I knew, I was eating low-calorie, whole-wheat bread with my sandwiches ALL OF THE TIME and liking it! In fact, I still eat it today, and so do my sons (e.g., toast, sandwiches, and hamburger buns). They don't know it is healthier or has less fat, and they don't need to!

Another time while grocery shopping I was struggling to find the whole milk I normally bought because the store now had so many different types of milk—skim, ½ percent, 1 percent, and 2 percent, as well as whole. On past diets I had tried skim milk with my cereal, but I couldn't get past the way it looks or the way it tastes. *Yuck!* I am a true cereal lover, but there was no way I was eating it with skim milk! The ½ percent milk looked too close to skim, so *"something"* said, *"Why not try the 1 percent?"* Much to my surprise, I loved it, and I have been drinking it ever since. Also, any time a recipe calls for milk **I ALWAYS** use 1 percent milk, and it is good too. As soon as my sons turned two, they were drinking 1 percent milk, and now no one knows the difference. I also started using 2 percent American cheese slices and shredded cheeses as stores began selling them. I have found that cutting calories and fat where you can makes a big difference over time.

Well, after a few weeks of learning to live with and enjoy these simple habits, of course there would be trouble in paradise. My boyfriend and I had a fight after I was not so nice to him, and *he decided* we should break up and just be friends. I was devastated, especially since I just knew, *in my mind*, that we were going to get married! So when my roommates left our apartment I spent a lot of time crying, but when they were around, I would go for really long walks. I would walk from one end of the campus to the other. As weeks passed, and we were no closer to getting back together, I reluctantly decided to accept whatever God's will was in the situation. However, while I waited I kept walking, and I found out that I love to walk.

I am not sure how many months passed from the time I replaced soda with water, regular white bread with low-fat, whole-wheat bread, whole milk with

1 percent milk, and a lifestyle of sitting around watching TV with recreational walking, but I would say it was probably about three months. However, because a lot was going on in my life it never occurred to me to check a scale or keep track of the time. *In my mind, nothing had changed…* Well, nothing except for a new lifestyle that gradually evolved. Shortly thereafter, something strange began to happen… I would see friends as I was out walking, and they would ask, *"Have you lost weight?"* I remember answering, *"I wish!"* However, one day one of my roommates saw me, and she said, *"You can lose weight, but don't try to blow away!"* She was implying that I was getting too skinny! How was that possible? *I thought I looked the same.*

A short while after this, I was sick and needed a ride to the clinic, so I called my ex. *After all, he did say that he would be there if I ever needed anything* **and** *we could still be friends.* So I used that as an excuse/reason to get my ride *and* to see him… Although I was sick, I still made sure I looked good when he picked me up. He said I looked nice, but his roommate, who came with him, said I looked *slimmer…* Hmmm… All of these people were commenting on my size and weight, but because I could still wear my regular clothes, I still *felt* like I weighed in the 150s. It wasn't until I went home for the holidays that I realized *"something"* had really happened. I just didn't notice until I went shopping with a friend, and I was picking up clothes that were 11/12s and 13/14s like I normally did, but they were all hanging off of me. At first I thought they were just cut big, so I asked the sales lady to bring me first a 9/10, then a 7/8 and then a 5/6! I was in total shock! *What was going on????*

What Really Happened?

I didn't know what was going on, but I was prancing around like you wouldn't believe! This was enough to finally make me get on a scale, which confirmed that I had indeed lost weight. I had gone from 152 pounds to 137 pounds in a matter of months, *without even realizing it!* It really felt like a miracle had taken place, and I just literally woke up one morning 15 pounds lighter, *just like I had prayed!* Was it a miracle, or did something else happen? *Would God have really answered my goofy prayer where I asked to just wake up one morning and have lost 15 pounds without dieting or any effort on my part?* As much as I wanted that to happen, it seemed ridiculous even to me.

I remember seeing someone from my neighborhood that barely recognized me. He said in amazement, "*Girl, you have lost all that weight!*" To him, and to others who had not seen me in a while, I had gone from the 160s (*remember the vending machine fiasco*) to 137. They were amazed by the results, and they wanted to know what happened. Well, because I didn't know, I couldn't tell them. The fact that I didn't have any answers made some ask if I was sick. After a few of those comments, a friend and I decided to go to the library to learn about AIDs because it had become a hot topic (*this was during the '80s*), and the only symptoms we knew of were people losing weight very quickly, without trying… Praise the Lord, that was not the case, but even I had to admit that my sudden weight loss was surprising even though I had been praying it would happen for years! Regardless, to the world, and to me, it seemed that I had miraculously lost a good deal of weight in a short amount of time, without dieting!

As I look back at that period, over the years and now, it is obvious that even though I did not go on a "diet," I did "*do something.*" Between the milk and bread changes and drinking more water than soda, I had significantly reduced my caloric and fat intake. By how much I don't know, because I did not, and do not to this day, count calories, but over time, it obviously made a huge difference. Also, by adding regular exercise (*walking*) to the picture, my metabolism changed, and I increased muscle while losing fat. So by listening to the little *voice* or *leading* that suggested I make small changes in the way I ate and acted (i.e., exercising and finding ways to combat stress, boredom, and loneliness that didn't involve food), I experienced major changes in my body—the way I looked and how I felt. There were also changes on a mental and emotional level as well…

Startling Revelations

One of the benefits of walking long distances is that you get a lot of time to think and reflect on your life and who you really are. By no means did I work out all of my issues and demons, but I did get an idea of who I was. *It was not always a pretty picture*, and I wanted to work on changing that… It is still an ongoing process, but the first step to solving a problem is recognizing that there is one. So I took that first step. Looking at the way I treated my ex, I knew I was wrong. I was too focused on what I wanted to achieve. Did I care what he wanted or what he needed? *No.* I only cared about keeping him and achieving the goals that I had set for my life. *He deserved better.* Coincidentally, after all of this self-reflection, we got back together. Isn't it interesting that once I began to understand, accept, and work on who I was, I found love? However, in what was probably less than five months, I was slim, I had my man back, I grew up quite a bit (*there was still work to be done*), my self-esteem was at an all-time high, and I learned valuable life-lessons on keeping my weight under control and being a better person.

Moving On & Keeping It Off

Not only did I take the weight off, but I kept it off as I finished college and moved to the Washington, D.C. area following my *future husband*. I left Augusta three days after graduation—it kind of felt like I was running away from home (*obviously I still had issues to work out*). However, I was very optimistic about the future. I was going to finally live my happily-ever-after! I was all set to reach my goal of getting married to a man with all of the qualities that I had prayed/asked for. It really didn't get any better than that! Well, in one respect, things did get even better as I managed to get down to 130 pounds right before the wedding!

I had not been that size since the sixth grade! So I was very slim (*some said too slim*) as I picked out my wedding gown, which was always my dream. I didn't have to diet or work to fit in the gown—*it just fit perfectly*. I believe this was mainly due to the fact that my lifestyle after college still included quite a bit of walking. Because I worked in downtown D.C., I enjoyed walking to see the sights during lunch, and because I didn't have a car, I walked to/from bus and train stations quite a bit. The water also remained a constant, and I limited snacks to one at work (maybe cookies from the vending machine) and one per evening (I was into chocolate doughnuts then, so I would eat one in bed at night with a whole bunch of water). I basically ate what I wanted, but I did it in moderation, and I kept on walking.

I should also mention that I stopped drinking alcohol of any kind during this time. I can't explain it other than to say that I just woke up one morning and realized that drinking had no purpose for me. As a result, I decided I would never drink again, *and I didn't*. This decision could be related to the fact that I was just really starting to take my Christian walk more seriously, but it could also be related to the fact that my father was an alcoholic, and I obviously know the dangers of overindulging. I can't really say why, but I just started to view drinking as a big, fat waste of time and calories, *and I still do*. Maybe I am ditzy enough sober! It is weird, but I don't even miss the taste of any of it. Aside from that, everything else pretty much stayed the same, and my weight stabilized around 137 (surprisingly, at this weight, my clothes are mostly a size 4 and 6), and that's where I stayed during the first year or so of my marriage.

Wake-Up Call #2
The Baby-Weight Battle
~ · ~ · ~ ~ · ~ · ~ · ~

By the second year of my marriage, my weight moved into the low 140s, which was OK because it kept me in my size 6 clothes. I still walked and ate reasonably, but just like everyone else, I had to work off a few pounds every now and then. However, I noticed a really cool benefit from the weight loss I experienced during my first wake-up call. My weight distribution and muscle tone improved to the point that even if I gained a few pounds and my weight crept into the mid/upper 140s, I could still wear the same clothes (*they were just a lot snugger than they needed to be*). So even when I had weight fluctuations, usually no one knew other than me and my husband. This is the main reason I don't like to let my weight go up more than a few pounds before I start working on it. By the time weight-gain is obvious to other people, it is exponentially harder to get it back under control. I can work off five pounds in private, which is how I prefer to handle it. So other than the occasional fluctuation (two to five pounds), my weight was pretty stable. Of course this would be the time when my husband and I would decide to start our family... *It was January of 1994, and I wanted a little boy for Christmas.*

Baby #1

I became pregnant with our first son in 1994, a few weeks sooner than I planned, and as during much of my adult life, I found myself anemic. I had just visited an ob/gyn to get prenatal vitamins, and she decided to do a pregnancy test just to make sure I wasn't already pregnant. Of course *I was already pregnant*, and while I was ecstatic to be on target for my "baby by Christmas" goal, I was exhausted and hungry until the prenatal vitamins kicked in. We were eating at *Denny's, Red Lobster, Chili's,* and *Taco Bell* on a regular basis, and I was asleep by 8:30 almost every night for the first three months. As a result, I gained eighteen pounds during the first trimester. Even as I grew less tired, I still had an *eating-good-time* throughout the pregnancy. When it was all said and done, I had gained forty-seven plus pounds (*I never got the final weigh-in because I went into labor a week early*). Praise the Lord, I had a healthy baby boy (9 pounds, 3.4 ounces)! We named him Christian because of a deal I made with God—*if He gave me a little boy by Christmas, I would name him Christian.* Well He did His part, so I did mine. I was ecstatic, but **I went home weighing 172 pounds!**

Of course this was alarming, but I didn't worry about it because for the first few weeks I was getting used to taking care of the baby. It was terrifying and tiring, but wonderful at the same time. However, around Christmas, about *a month after having the baby*, my husband *carefully* asked if I wanted my Christmas gifts to be bought in a size 6 *or* the size I was at the time (*who knows what that was*). This was the first thought I had about my weight and my future plans concerning it. I have to admit I expected to lose more weight during the delivery. It never occurred to me that I would come home in the 170s. However, my husband's question forced me to make a key decision that affected my thinking forever...

After much thought and deliberation, *I chose the size 6 clothes* even though it seemed ridiculous at the time. I did agree to accept a few jackets in larger sizes because I was breastfeeding, and I could not squeeze "*my new friends*" into size 6 or 8 jackets. However, it was very important for me not to have skirts, dresses, or pants in larger sizes. I wanted to be forced to get back into my normal clothes. *I didn't want a closet full of clothes in temporary sizes.* Not saying that I would never buy a larger size depending on how clothes are cut because I would be lying, but I mean I don't want my closet to be filled with clothes in many varying sizes that I can't wear. For the most part, I want to wear the same clothes for years, as long as they are fashionable, of course. I don't want "*heavy*" clothes versus "*slim*" clothes. I just want to be able to wear the same shorts, sundresses, or swimsuits next year if I still like them. I don't want to ever be locked into buying something to wear each season. I wanted my old body back! For all of these reasons, *I decided* then and there that, no matter what, I was going to continue wearing clothes in the same size! *As I am sure you know, this is easier said than done...*

Because I was breastfeeding and going for walks with my son in the stroller, I was down to about 164 pounds after about six weeks, which I felt was a major accomplishment. Of course this would be about the time I received a wonderful assortment of Christmas presents, which included *pants and skirts, all in a size 6.* When my husband wasn't around I tried on the beautiful slacks he had picked out, but I could not even come close to fastening them because the sides of the pants had almost six inches of space between them! Oh, I was a size 6 alright—*six inches away from being able to fasten my pants!* I could also squeeze into the new skirts, but again the sides had inches of room that kept me from even thinking about trying to fasten them. I also tried on some of my old clothes, but it was the same story—I was definitely nowhere close to being a size 6! Even with this disappointing dose of reality, I wasn't too discouraged, as I focused on a reasonable short-term goal of just trying to see any number in the 150s.

~·~·~· A Long, Hard Road ·~·~·~

The biggest lesson I learned about losing baby-weight is that you can eat like you are crazy while you are pregnant, but once you have the baby, you have to start eating like you have some sense again, *REAL QUICK*. Otherwise, you will be walking around with the same baby fat years later! I also learned that you have to start exercising as soon as you are able to, which is why I also asked for a treadmill for Christmas. The treadmill was a good idea, but there was still way too much late-night eating going on… Because my husband never said anything negative about the *Chip Ahoy* cookies I ate during the night while I breastfed the baby, I kept on eating lots of them. What a cop-out! I knew better, and I soon learned better because the caffeine from the chocolate kept the baby awake. Also, because my husband was "helping with the cooking," we were eating more meals than we normally would from *Kentucky Fried Chicken*. On top of that, I was struggling to regain control over my *chocoholic* tendencies, and I had started scarfing down at least ten miniature *Reese's Peanut Butter Cups* at a time or polishing off a pack of *Keebler Fudge Covered Graham Crackers* in a day. I might also drink a twenty-ounce soda in the evening.

Because of these eating habits, I was still in the 160s by the time the baby reached three months, yet I had the nerve to ask God, "Why?" However, a comment my mother made after seeing me go upstairs with a handful of *Reese's Cups* actually helped wake me up. She said in her usual Southern accent, "*You need to lay off of that old chocolate!*" Then it seems again that "something" said, "*She's right, and while you are at it, you should stop drinking sodas and going to Kentucky Fried Chicken until you get out of the 160s.*" That was so hard because I had grown to love the *Original Recipe* drumsticks.

Well, I listened to both suggestions and added a combination of walking and light running on the treadmill five days a week to my routine. I started with ten minutes while the baby was napping or in the swing, and each day I went a little farther, even if it was just a minute longer or an extra tenth of a mile. Eventually I got up to about forty minutes of mostly jogging five days a week. I also walked all over the neighborhood and/or mall with my son in his stroller almost every day. He loved being outside and seeing sights, which was a major plus. For my first Mother's Day gift I asked for rollerblades and gear. I then took a class and started skating for fun and exercise. My husband and I would take the baby to the park, and I would skate. As a result, I was back in my old clothes before he turned five months, and within a few weeks after that I was in the low 140s, which is the highest weight I ever want to be.

Baby # 2

I enjoyed being back at this weight for about a year when "we" decided that it was a good time to plan another pregnancy. This time I was already taking prenatal vitamins so I did not get anemic, but I still ate any and everything I wanted. I loved being pregnant! However, for the first time I experienced nausea. I never vomited, but I felt yuck at different times during the day. After crackers and ginger ale didn't work, I found that huge sandwiches of eggs, bacon, and/or sausage *with ketchup* helped combat my nausea. It was so yummy! Because I was still at home with my first son, I was able to make large breakfasts that consisted of three jumbo eggs and four thick slices of bacon—sometimes I even added two pork sausage patties. I was being so greedy, *but it was so good!* For some reason the combination of eggs, bacon, sausage, and ketchup made the nausea go away immediately, and I felt great. So anytime I felt queasy I would make one of these sandwiches no matter what time of the day or night!

I have to tell you, I must have eaten about a thousand eggs during this pregnancy, and I am not exaggerating! Fortunately my doctor said cholesterol was not an issue while I was pregnant, but she did say that the excessive egg/bacon/sausage eating needed to go away as soon as I had the baby. By the end of the pregnancy I had gained forty plus pounds. Again, I missed the final weigh-in because a Cesarean was scheduled a week before the due date (the baby was breach). I did not gain as much as during the first pregnancy, which was probably due to the fact that I was more active. I even remember playing kickball with some kids during my seventh month. However, in spite of that small lapse in judgment, I was blessed with another healthy baby boy who weighed 9 pounds, 7.8 ounces! Even though I just knew I was having a little girl for Christmas this time, I was thrilled because I always wanted two sons to carry on my husband's family name—this one just came sooner than I expected! We were all very happy with little Evan's arrival, but the battle to get my weight back under control was on yet AGAIN.

Round Two

I don't even remember how much I weighed when I came home this time. I think I was too punch-drunk. I was recovering from a Cesarean, which was a little more intense physically. The whole *don't-lift-more-than-twenty-pounds* rule was a little hard to adjust to when I already had a twenty-five plus pound bundle of joy at home waiting for me to pick him up! Another adjustment was not being able to take the stairs as much, especially when our house was filled with them. I definitely had more on my mind this time, as I didn't want my first son to feel displaced or resentful toward the new baby. However, because my attention was divided, the breastfeeding adjustment was not as easy as it had been the first time, so I had to spend extra time getting both of us used to it. Also, because the boys were so close in age, they were both in diapers at the same time! It certainly was a lot to juggle, so I think my weight was the last thing on my mind!

As you can imagine, after I got home from the hospital I didn't want any eggs for a *long* time. I find it funny now that Evan rarely eats eggs unless they are on a sandwich with bacon/sausage and ketchup! However, for me the jumbo eggs and bacon sandwiches were a thing of the past. I went back to cereal and 1 percent milk for breakfast as well as peanut butter and jelly sandwiches on low-fat, whole-wheat bread and fruit or a plain, baked sweet potato for lunch during the week. Visits to fast-food restaurants were cut down to a minimum, as I had learned my lesson from the first pregnancy.

Because of the Cesarean, I started off with short walks in our neighborhood until I felt stronger. By the time the baby was six weeks old, and after receiving my doctor's approval, I was back on the treadmill following the same routine I did after having my first son. However, this time I also added walks with the kids in their double stroller (*one of the world's greatest inventions*). When it was cold we walked in the mall, and when it was warm, we walked around the neighborhood or downtown D.C. They both loved riding the subway and seeing sights, so I would take them all over the place, walking to my heart's content. I also continued to rollerblade. All of this activity, combined with drinking mostly water and very little soda, got me off to a good start. *However…*

A Rude Awakening

I was stuck at 158 for a long while, and I started to wonder what was causing the lengthy plateau. OK, I will admit that I was still indulging in chocolate way too often, probably because I felt a little overwhelmed in the beginning. I stayed at home with both of the boys for the first four months, which is easier in some ways (e.g., *you don't have to pack them up every morning to go to a daycare*), but harder in others (e.g., *you are the primary caregiver morning, noon, and night as well as the clean-up crew*). Obviously I was still adjusting, but I was pooped, which is probably why I found myself overeating at night. Even though I wasn't hungry, I found myself in a hard-to-stop eating frenzy where I might eat a *few* cookies, and then a *few* chips and then maybe a twenty-ounce soda. It wasn't that I was craving these foods, but when I eat too many sweets, I usually get a bad taste in my mouth, which makes me want to eat something salty to get rid of the taste. Then, of course, thirst kicks in… Thus the cycle of late-night overeating began, leaving me feeling guilty and yuck! So this was definitely an area I had to get under control, but there was also the matter of how much I was eating during the day…

My big "Aha" moment (*as Oprah would say*) happened one day when my stepdaughter, who was ten at the time, saw me eating a big bowl of Captain Crunch cereal for breakfast. She didn't comment on the first bowl, but when I filled up, *and I do mean filled up*, a second bowl, she said, "You must be *really* hungry!" Of course I looked at her and said, " *What do you mean?*"What was wrong with getting a refill of cereal, for Pete's sake??? Cereal is healthy! Well, probably nothing if the bowl was not huge, *but it was*, and if the first serving wasn't a full one, *but it was*. I am sure a range of emotions crossed my face as her words sank in: *annoyance, embarrassment, shock, etc*… This was the first time I ever took time to think about not just what I was eating, but about *how much*. I knew nothing was wrong with eating cereal, especially since I was using 1 percent milk! Cereal is a good thing, but *was I eating too much of it????*

To say the least, I was caught off guard by the innocent question of a child. However, after sulking and thinking about it over the next few days, I finally accepted that I really wasn't hungry enough for that second bowl of cereal, and I really didn't need to use such big bowls in the first place. I was really eating more out of habit and taste than hunger. As a result, I decided not to eat more than one *normal-size* bowl of cereal for breakfast. Then I started to look at lunch and dinner to see if I could find other examples of my overeating. *You know there were...* It is amazing how we often eat without thinking, but as soon as we spend some time *honestly* thinking about what we are eating and how much, it becomes easier to make changes. Cutting down on portion sizes still allowed me to eat what I wanted, but I now ate it like I had some sense. In addition to the other modifications (e.g., reducing soda consumption to once/twice a week, laying off of the chocolate, hitting the treadmill like before, walking the kids all over the place, etc.) this was enough to help me get out of the 150s again. A few months later I was back in my size 6 clothes again. *Praise the Lord, I had won the baby-weight battle a second time*! It wasn't easy, but it definitely can be done.

~

Wake-Up Call #3
The Spinning Out of Control Phase
~ • ~ • ~ ~ • ~ • ~ • ~

Even though my husband and I have made a conscious decision that we don't want to have any more children (our sons are fifteen and thirteen now), it still requires a *conscious* effort for me to stay the same size year after year. I'd be lying if I didn't say that along the way there are times when I struggle with eating too much and exercising too little. I find that this is more likely to happen when my life is out of balance or when I work in corporate environments where the workload is crazy and there is a whole lot of sitting. I found myself in this situation a few years ago when I was a manager at a large telecommunications company.

Because my job was so hectic, I usually worked through lunch and spent hours on my laptop at night. Also, because we lived in a neighborhood that didn't have sidewalks, trails, or paths, **and** we got home so late, we rarely walked or spent time outside during the week. This was around the time that I wrote my first book and was trying to promote it. The boys were small, my stepdaughter lived with us, and my husband had a long commute into Washington, D.C. As a result, pick-ups/drop-offs, daytime school events, doctors' appointments and shopping trips for the children, cooking, and homework were usually my domain. Who had time for exercise or to pay attention to what I was eating? *I was beyond exhausted!*

Unfortunately I didn't realize how crazy my life had become until I started having heart palpitations. After extensive tests and having to wear a Holter monitor (*tracks heart activity*), I found out that I was severely anemic, which was affecting my heart. Even though I had been anemic over the years, the doctor wanted to hear about my schedule/lifestyle. So I confessed to staying up many nights working until 2:00 a.m., and I woke up at 6:00 a.m. He also wanted to know about my eating habits... I had strayed considerably from many of the good habits I had before—I had stopped eating low-fat, low-calorie bread, and I began snacking on sweets, chips, and sodas whenever I felt like it. I guess I was so busy trying to take care of everyone else and working that I was not doing a very good job of taking care of myself... So I wasn't surprised when the doctor told me that I needed more rest, more iron, and better eating habits. He said the peanut butter and jelly I was eating for lunch was OK, but not for *EVERY* day. He recommended I take supplements and eat iron-rich foods like roast beef occasionally. *I agreed.*

This was all good advice, but the part about "not eating peanut butter and jelly every day" had an adverse affect. I had to eat, and the fixings for peanut butter and jelly could be easily kept at work and ready to eat without much fuss or thought. However, without it, I was left wondering what to eat for lunch... *Not good!* I was confused and hungry in the midst of a chaotic work and family schedule, which led me to start asking people to bring me lunch back from restaurants when they went out (e.g., *Taco Bell*, *Popeyes*, etc.). Somehow I don't think this is what the doctor had in mind when he told me to vary my diet! So as I struggled to deal with my crazy schedule and life in general, my weight started to creep back into the 150s.

What's Done In The Dark...
The weight came on so gradually that I thought I was actually getting away with the extra eating. I could still wear the same clothes, so I was able to delude myself for a while. In fact, I convinced myself that I wasn't really eating that much. Have you noticed that when your life gets crazy, it feels really good to eat in the bed and watch TV after your work is finished and your kids are asleep? I have to tell you that during this time it felt *REAL* good to me! Since I had given up chocolate candy and cookies during Wake-up Call #2, I ate ice cream,

caramel, and other sweet treats instead. I remember asking my husband to bring me seconds on my cup of ice cream as I sat in bed going through the massive amounts of e-mails from work. Unfortunately, things got even worse during the summer… My cousin got me to try an *Oreo*, even though I told her I was a recovering chocoholic. She looked skeptical and said, "*One won't hurt.*"

I really should have known better. The next thing you know I was eating *Oreos* like they were going out of style! They just *seemed* to speak to what was ailing me, and instead of crying and acknowledging that the pace of my life was not working, *I ate Oreos…* This foolishness went on for a few months, and *I do mean foolishness.* Anytime there was a sale on *Oreos* (minis or full-sized), I would load up. I ate them at work, in the car, and at home. I could not believe it, but I had developed an *Oreo habit!* After a while, the *evidence* of "my habit" became noticeable. I remember looking down in the shower and when I wore certain sweater outfits, and my thighs were the first thing I saw. *They were definitely sticking out more in the front!* I then started to notice that most of my clothes were extremely tight. In fact, I had to stand up super straight, with my stomach sucked in for my normal clothes to even fit comfortably. The changes were really starting to bother me, especially when I went home to Georgia to visit my family. The whole time I was there I was so self-conscious and uncomfortable in my *very snug* clothes.

However, the final straw did not happen until I went to a family gathering back in Virginia, where I wore a pair of snug-fitting jeans, which *I thought* were hidden by a long jacket. I casually mentioned that I had put on a few pounds, and one of my relatives overheard and immediately said, "I *thought you were looking a little hippy!*" I looked at her for a moment, trying not to let my anger and hurt show. I didn't like being called "*hippy,*" and doggone it, I was tired of having to constantly suck in my stomach tightly just to fit into my clothes. So I decided it was time to get serious about my life *and* my weight.

<u>Waking Up To Smell the Coffee</u>
My first step toward getting serious was finally allowing myself to have the long, private cry I had been on the verge of for months. Even though I had beautiful, healthy children, a great husband, a beautiful house in a nice area, a

"*good*" job where I had just received the best performance evaluation I had ever gotten, and I had been recommended for a senior management position, I was forced to admit that *I wasn't happy*. To be honest, my life was just moving way too fast… *I literally could not keep up*. I was always rushing to do something (e.g., pick up kids, grocery shop, cook, soccer practices, field trips, doctor's appointments, laundry, help with homework, finish my work, etc.). I was always rushing the kids. We were living right up to our means and beyond financially. There were so many expectations I was trying to meet at work, and I had personal goals I was trying to reach as well. There was always just so doggone much to do. I often wondered, "*How did my life turn into this crazy existence?*"

During this time my husband used to jokingly refer to my laptop as my "boyfriend" because I was on it working past 1:00 a.m. many nights. However, the jokes were not funny to me as I would often get fifty to sixty plus new e-mails a day at work, and I was expected to either address them or have knowledge of them when I least expected it. This was extremely stressful for me because, as I said before, I am not the most technically gifted person in the world. In fact, a lot of what I learned about managing an analysis and design team was learned on the fly. *I certainly didn't know how to do most of it before I got the job.* In fact, I was so inexperienced that when the company first gave me a laptop I thought it was a blessing, but I slowly came to realize that it was a way for them to get me to work more—*after hours, when I was home with a sick child and even when I was sick.* I remember working on employee performance reviews while I was at home with strep throat. I guess that was somewhat of a break.

I was slowly losing it though. In fact, I recall laughing hysterically one evening when my husband asked me the last time I had mopped the kitchen. I was like, "*I don't know,*" and in my mind, I was thinking, "*I don't care either.*" **I really didn't.** We had three finished levels, and it was major work just to keep it *somewhat* clean. Also, we had an acre lot, but I hate to do yard work, and I was so busy with work that we rarely invited anyone over, so I often wondered why did we need it all? It was definitely more work than it was enjoyment, and it was all just too much for me at that point—*the job, my ambitions, the house, living right up to our means* (e.g., huge mortgage, private school for two kids, etc.) *the wife role, the kids…*

As a result, my physical appearance (*mainly my weight*) and my overall health began to reflect my inner turmoil. I loved my family and the things we had acquired, but something really needed to change… During that time I could clearly see how some people can be fooled into thinking they want a divorce. Although I have never wanted one, I can certainly understand how wanting a life change can cause someone to mistakenly think that his or her spouse is the problem when really it could be what my husband likes to call a "smokescreen." You may be tired or frustrated about your job or the amount of running around you do as a parent, cooking, cleaning, financial struggles, not enough time as a couple, not enough time as a person, and sometimes you could mistakenly think that your spouse is the problem. However, the "problem" could really be *you* or how complicated you and your spouse have allowed your lives to become. I know for us many of our own choices had complicated our lives (e.g., a larger house than we needed, the decision to hold onto properties and deal with the headaches of being landlords, etc.), and my husband and I both experienced the frustration caused by these *complications*.

This was back in 2001, and it was about the time that many telecommunications companies started to cut back, and as a result, layoffs became pretty commonplace. I went from managing a team of thirteen people to a team of less than six in a few months, and the rumblings about further budget cuts were a source of concern for almost everyone around me. I'd be lying if I didn't say that with the mortgage we had and all of our other financial obligations, the thought of being laid off was pretty frightening. However, the more I thought about it, the more I realized that we always have options… Although I loved my house and my lot, was holding on to it and the job it required more important than my quality of life? Could I be just as happy living in the three-level townhouse I used to love, thereby simplifying my life for a time so I could breathe and think clearly? I started to think back to the first home we ever bought. We were so happy there… *In fact, I never wanted to leave it in the first place.* It was in a neighborhood where I enjoyed walking to the grocery store, restaurants, and to the post office. I thought about how much our kids would enjoy walking to the playgrounds and the pool. Because I had been so busy with work and we lived in a neighborhood without a pool, they hadn't even learned to swim. We rarely had time to go to the pool, but what if I changed things? *Maybe we would have time then… Maybe*

I could enjoy the kids and my husband with a clear, stress-free mind. Maybe I could enjoy some time to myself and get back to the long walks I had been missing. I certainly needed the clarity that long walks usually helped to bring...

Exit Strategy

As I started having these thoughts I suddenly felt calmer about everything, and I spent more time thinking about what was truly important to me—*family, health,* **and** *quality of life,* not a job or house that seemed impressive on the surface. This is especially funny now as I remember a time when a family member came over to our house for dinner, and she commented that we had *arrived* (based on our house, I guess). *Arrived?* How was it possible that we had *arrived* when I felt trapped by my job, the upkeep of my house, and our financial obligations? I was tired, and I was not as happy as I thought I would be... So wherever it was that we had *arrived,* I didn't want to be! I wanted to walk away from the things in my life that had me feeling like someone had placed me in a chokehold. I could get a similar/better house in the future, but *at the right time, under the right circumstances,* without the pressure cooker environment. I *like* having nice things, but I **value** peace of mind, and I was immediately more at peace as I started to imagine my life without the job and the material things that tied me to it. I remember being excited as I looked forward to the possibility of a different life, one with less tension and stress. A life that was not as rushed...

So when the executives at my company started talking about layoffs, I remember getting very excited once I found out that I could get a substantial amount of money to walk away. Based on the information I received, I worked up the courage to go home and ask my husband if I could *volunteer* for the layoff/ severance package... We could sell our house and go back to our old townhouse and a much simpler life, where we could regroup and enjoy our lives and children a bit. We could also sell our other house and get out of the landlord business for a while. To the world, I know we looked crazy. I also know it was hard on my husband because he put his blood, sweat, and tears into getting the house built, but he agreed. I was so glad he did because I desperately needed time and clarity to get myself on the right path so I could put our relationship back in its proper place... *It hadn't been for a while, and I didn't like that...* I no longer wanted the laptop to be my boyfriend. *In fact, I realized that I needed more quality time with him and my family in general.* My work/desire for more had taken over, and the result had left our lives out of balance. *I could not allow it to continue...*

Moving Forward

As we discussed putting the house on the market and considered our move, the kids were actually happy—my oldest son was excited about the pool/basketball courts, and my youngest son was happy to go to the public school's half-day kindergarten. The move would allow me to enjoy some much needed one-on-one time with him, where we could work and play together without being rushed. It is funny how this worked out because I had been feeling guilty that he never got the one-on-one time with me that his brother had because I went back to work when he was four months old. However, this could be *our* special time, and I was looking forward to it.

Another perk was that I could be home when my oldest son came home from school so we could review homework *BEFORE* dinner. Maybe we could even eat dinner before 7:00! *Also, maybe I wouldn't have to rush from work to pick him up, where he would have to change in the car on the way to soccer practice, and I would more than likely be on a conference call while I watched and then race home to make dinner, eat, look over everyone's homework/work with them, rush them to take a bath, get them in bed, get out the ice cream and my laptop, and begin tackling e-mails from work until the wee hours of the morning!* It was crazy. It is no wonder I was having heart palpitations and had no time for my husband or myself!

Even though the craziness and the *busyness* of my life helped me to see clearly that I was ready to make this major change, I must admit it was pretty hard for me to leave on many levels... I was still that little girl who grew up in the projects and always dreamt of living in a house like the one I was leaving. We were in the *right* house, in the *right* area, but at the *wrong* time and definitely under the *wrong* circumstances. **I knew the house had to go!** However, there were some who thought we were crazy to leave, but that was OK because I don't think they understood that this beautiful house tied me to a job that I hated and a lifestyle I no longer wanted...

I know there were others who found it even crazier that I would leave a job where I was probably just one step away from a senior management position. I was well-respected and decently paid, but to get over the next hurdle, I knew I would need to work even harder than I already was. How was I going to do that? *I was already too tired to do what I was currently doing!* Also, with the number of people that had been let go already, the people who stayed behind would obviously have to take on even more responsibility. For me that was a scary prospect as I was already a manager and a business analyst—I managed other analysts, making sure they had what they needed to do their jobs and that they did it well. I was also responsible for doing the work of an analyst myself. Because I had been doing all of this so well (*I had the reviews, awards and bonuses to prove it*), I started to realize that I was probably not going to be selected for a layoff. Based on my performance, I was *a perfect candidate for the company to keep around and over work*. I don't know if I ever shared this revelation with my husband, but I really felt it was the case. If I didn't tell him, it could have been because I worried about our future if I stayed... Could my sanity take more work than I had already been doing? *What toll would it have on our marriage and family life?*

If I stayed I would have to commit to doing an excellent job at whatever work that came my way, as I don't like to fail or look like a boob. How would I continue to perform at a level of excellence at work and at home, stay healthy and keep my sanity? It was already getting harder to leave *work* at work, especially for a woman who likes to *autograph her work with excellence* and to compete. Because of this self-motivation/torment my mind was always on what was going to come up next: *How many new e-mails would I get? What new projects would I be assigned to? How much more time would be shaved off of our deliverables schedule (meaning we would have to do more, faster)? What new standards would be imposed on our deliverables, causing us to have to do more work to accomplish the same tasks? How many more analysts would we lose?*

I remember walking on the beach during a vacation with my family, and I found myself struggling to get my mind off of the latest crisis I was facing at work. Crazy, huh? *The sad thing was that I could not silence the work-related noise in my mind.* My thoughts were totally consumed. I am not sure what a nervous breakdown is, but I could have been on the verge of one. Although I know many people who handle this type of stress on a daily basis with style and efficiency, *I am not one of those people. This level of stress coupled with a family was just too much for me.*

Going For It

I don't know when I was done deliberating on whether to stay or go, but there came a point where I just knew I was done. One day at work I remember humming the lyrics from and joking about two radically different songs that captured the essence of what I was feeling: 1) A country song by Johnny Paycheck that I heard during my childhood, "*Take this job and shove it, I ain't working here no more…*"; and 2) A rap song by DMX (I heard it in the movie *Like Mike*), "*Ya'll gonna make me lose my mind up in here, up in here… Ya'll gonna make me act a fool up in here, up in here… Ya'll gonna make me lose my cool up in here, up in here…*" Although I jokingly sang these lyrics as the work drove me crazy, there was an edge of truth and sometimes a little hysteria mixed in with the jokes. *It was time to go…*

Even though leaving a "good" job when I was not in danger of being laid off seemed crazy, I was beyond caring. I was tired and burnt out just from being a manager, so why on earth was I even trying to become a senior manager? I never even wanted to be in management in the first place! However, I was just so flattered by the praise and bonuses, and I wanted to see what it was like to be in management. However, I never expected to ever even be near a senior management level so soon… Did that mean that one day I could be a director if I wanted? Tempting, but did I even want that? For a time I was confused, but *not anymore.*

I wanted, and desperately needed, time to re-evaluate my life and the direction in which I was headed. Looking back at this period, I clearly understand how people wind up having high blood pressure, heart attacks, ulcers, drinking/drug addictions, weight problems, marital troubles/divorce, neglected/unsupervised children, etc… The *weight* of what we allow our lives to become can take a heavy toll on us if we let things spiral out of control. I felt my life spiraling out of control, but I wanted to stop it while there was time and before any irreparable damage was done. I was thankful that after my husband got over the initial shock, he finally gave me his blessing to volunteer for the layoff. I give him a lot of credit because I know how much he loved our old house, as well as the tremendous effort he put into building it. Also, the pretty decent salary I earned was hard to walk away from. However, I needed to spend more quality time with our children and slow things down a bit... We sold the house shortly thereafter, and I walked away with a nice severance package, as well as unemployment benefits for a year (an unexpected surprise), which gave me some much needed time off. *This was the perfect time to take a break and rethink the direction and pace of my life.*

A Fresh Start

Now that the pace of my life was a little slower I finally had time to look in the mirror and focus on the shape I was in and try to deal with it. I was back in the 150s, and yet again, I realized I did not want to go out like this. *This was not who I am.* I had to get myself together. It was obvious that I needed to change my lifestyle so that we were more physically active as a family, and I needed to improve my eating habits to get back to a healthier weight and to make sure I didn't wind up anemic again. I also wanted to be comfortable in my clothes again. So my husband and I decided to join a new gym nearby. I was really excited because *I actually had time to go*, and the membership included an evaluation from a trainer to determine my body mass index (BMI) and fitness goals. I also got a few free hours with the trainer, which I loved because I had always wanted a personal trainer. He determined that my main goals should be to reduce my BMI and improve my core strength, so I was excited to get things rolling.

I started my new regimen by showing my trainer, *a muscle-bound guy who seemed to know what he was doing*, pictures of how I wanted my new body to look (e.g., *I had a picture of Naomi Campbell's midsection and Donna Richardson's arms, etc.*). The only constraint I had was that I did not want to increase the size of my calves—they could be more toned, maybe even leaner, but *no bulk could be added.* My calves have always been very developed, even as a child. People used to ask if I ran track or played tennis, but my answer has always been that my calves are just big. *End of story.* So I showed the trainer pictures of models with *toned, lean legs*, not bulky, overly muscular ones. Aside from this one area, I came with an open mind, and I was ready to get in the best shape of my life.

Based on my goals and pictures, the trainer came up with a routine where I would eat six small meals a day and combine a moderate amount of cardio activity (e.g., stair climber, treadmill, elliptical machine, etc.) with weight training. I was also instructed to eat a protein snack before my workouts (e.g., almonds or a slice of luncheon meat, etc.). Even though I did not want to increase the size of my calf muscles, my weight training routine still included the use of a free-weight machine that worked this area. I was suspicious and so was my husband (*he was skeptical all along and tried to warn me, but of course I didn't listen to him*), but the trainer seemed knowledgeable so I faithfully followed his regimen. *Even when he said I should not weigh myself for the first three months...*

I was just so excited to have time to focus on myself that some days I even went to the gym twice a day. On the second visit, I would swim or just walk on the treadmill. Even though all of this activity kept me busy, I was diligent about keeping a log of my activities as the trainer suggested so I could monitor my progress. I can't tell you how thrilled I was about my new regimen and how my body was going to change. I already felt better physically and emotionally, and I was determined to get as physically fit as I could. As I worked toward this goal, I struggled with one thing in particular—*the trainer's admonition not to weigh myself for the first few months*. His reasoning was that I might not see actual weight loss as fat was being replaced by muscle. So I continued on for the next few weeks, but I couldn't wait to see some sort of progress or results! I wanted to see *something* after weeks of hard work. Well, after about six weeks of hard work, I saw something alright—*a pointy bulge at the top of my calves*!

I literally lost it! ***THIS WAS THE ONE THING I TOLD HIM I DID NOT WANT!*** The workout regimen he prescribed obviously worked my calf muscles way too much, and, as I said *repeatedly*, the last thing I needed was to increase my calf size! So being the distrustful person that I am, I began to question *everything* he had told me to do, and he lost most of his credibility in my eyes. *Why didn't I listen to my husband?* He warned me to be careful with the weight training because I could wind up bulking up instead of slimming down like I wanted. *Why did I listen to that trainer?* He obviously could not be trusted! However, before I totally lost my mind and went off the deep end, I decided to get on a scale to see if there was anything positive I could find to restore my faith in the trainer and his prescribed path for me, *minus the leg exercises of course*. Imagine my surprise when I found out that I had not lost any weight. In fact, I had **gained** almost eight pounds! I can't tell you how mad I was after spending so much time and money at that gym and eating those six little meals to find myself in the 160s again. I didn't care if some of it was muscle! I was so mad that I stopped going to the gym completely!

Taking Matters into My Own Hands

Once I went through the full range of emotions from rage to sadness (*I cried*) to apathy, I had a revelation... I could get better results than this on my own, and I had as I worked to get off baby-weight in the past. *How soon we forget...* So instead of the regimen I had been following, I decided to go back to my "normal" meals (i.e., cereal and 1 percent milk for breakfast, a sandwich and fruit for lunch, and a reasonable dinner of a meat, two vegetables, and bread) and snacks (e.g., fruit during the day and limited sweets after dinner, etc.). However, there were a few new rules: *no eating after 9:00 p.m. (I wanted to say 8:00, but I needed to ease into it)*; *no more chocolate or cookies until I could get my snacking under control (I was/still am a recovering chocoholic); sodas were for special occasions; drink water 90 percent of the time*; and only *eat meals out of hunger*, which was three meals a day, **not six**. Instead of going back to the gym, I started going for long walks to the post office, bank, grocery store, and school with my sons—they rode their scooters, and I walked or jogged after them. When they were in school I still walked out of necessity or just for fun. *Wasn't this one of the reasons why I moved back to this neighborhood in the first place?* I had completely forgotten as I got caught up in the gym/trainer routine.

On the weekends I also enjoyed running behind the boys as they rode their bicycles and scooters, and we would often stop at the playground to play basketball or kickball (*I played the field while they kicked and ran*—this is actually a great workout). As a family we also went to parks where my husband and I would throw the Frisbee or play baseball or soccer with them. So basically I created my own exercise routine that consisted of lots of walking and playing with my kids. They enjoyed the extra attention, we strengthened our bond as a family, and something surprising happened. I was back in the low 140s within a few months, *without* going to the gym and *without* starving myself! Guess what else? I was able to go back to Georgia "comfortably" wearing my clothes and not sucking in my gut at all times, and I felt better than I had in years. I was amazed because the new regimen/routine I had adopted felt very easy and practical.

Some of the people who saw me during my earlier "*hippy*" visit wanted to know my secret for getting the weight off. What I shared with them and have described in this wake-up call is an oversimplified explanation (*the detailed, albeit simple, one can be found in Chapters 7 and 8*) of all of the practices I implemented and continue to revisit at the first sign of trouble today. I decided to write this book because I have never seen anything on the market that ever made eating better and losing weight sound easy or practical. What I did really felt too easy, and even I was surprised at how quickly I lost the weight. *The good news is that what I did can be varied and tailored to work for you as well.*

The Last Laugh

When I returned to Virginia, I finally saw the relative who made the "hippy" comment, and the first thing she did was comment on my weight loss, but this time she said I had gotten too skinny! I had to laugh at this one because I was around 140 pounds (*based on my height and bone structure, this puts me in size 6 and 4 clothes, depending on the store*), but now I was too skinny! So I had gone from being "hippy" to "too skinny" in a matter of months! *This is why you should never base your body image on what others think of you—it should be based on your health and how you feel about yourself.* As this relative kept pressing the "too skinny" point, she then wanted to know how I had lost the weight. So I shared some of the habits I just described in this chapter. Still not satisfied, she wanted to know what was going to happen when I returned to my old eating habits.

I was annoyed by this point, but I told her that the habits and practices I now follow are a way of life, *not a diet*. So even if I stray temporarily (e.g., during vacations, stressful times, etc.), I can always find my way back because the habits are not hard to follow once you get used to them. Also, in the long run, they will keep me healthy, and I love the fact that I don't have to look for the latest diet book or regimen to get back on track in times of trouble. *I know what to do.* At this point in my life, I feel like I really know my body and what works to keep it at a healthy weight, and that is very empowering. *I want you to feel that same sense of power and control where your weight is concerned, because I know you can.*

Even though I have really enjoyed being back in a size 6 and being able to have the last laugh on the "hippy" incident, the best outcome from this wake-up call was the fact that it put me on a path that keeps family and quality of life first. So although my life has changed over the years, I have learned that *we have the power to chart our own course.* However, we sometimes may need a wake-up call(s) to do this. This is why I decided to share mine and the lessons I learned from them. I am sure you have had your own, but you may not have had a chance to devise a plan to get from *where you are* to *where you want to be.* The remaining chapters of this book are designed to help you do just that—go from Point **A** *(where you* **Are)** to Point **B** *(where you want to* **Be).** The lessons I learned from living through the events I just shared changed my life, and I believe they can change yours too. I really believe you can do it, so now all that is left is for you to get started. You have definitely heard more than enough about me, so now let's turn our attention to **you**...

∾

Chapter 4

Regroup & Recover (Step 2)

So, are you getting a better idea of who you are and who you want to be? *Have you remembered the person that you thought you'd become or that you always wanted to be?* I surely hope so because that person is on the inside of you kicking, screaming, and scratching to get out so you can live life to the fullest. You don't believe me? Well why do you think many of us experience so much inner turmoil? *Because there is conflict between the person we have allowed ourselves to become and the person we always wanted to be.* Well enough of that! **Life is too short for you not to consciously work to be who you want to be.**

We can all be *who* and *what* we want to be if we *decide what we want and commit to change.* However, before we can successfully do this, we need to figure a few things out first:

- Where Do You Start?
- Assess Where You Are & Make A Commitment To Change…
- What's *Eating* You?

This is why step two of my *Healthy Weight for Life®* program is for you to *Regroup & Recover*… You already began the work of understanding *how* you got to where you are today in the last chapter, but now it is time for you to *regroup*. In other words, acknowledge the truths/facts (e.g., your weight, BMI, cholesterol or blood pressure readings, worrisome symptoms, etc.) that you might have hidden from in the past. It is time to get everything out in the open as it relates to your physical self, so you can come up with a plan for how you will move forward. Don't get me wrong, the mental/emotional aspects are extremely important, but you must be armed with the necessary physical information before you can be sufficiently motivated to move forward.

With that said, even with this information, you won't get far until you deal with one of the biggest and most critical components of the whole plan—the point where you determine what's eating you and *recover* from it once and for all. Unfortunately so much of the focus is on *what* you are eating, but hardly anyone ever focuses on "*what is eating you.*" What feelings have you suppressed? What stress or issues aren't you dealing with? *What truth are you running from?* That is the million-dollar question—*What's eating you?* Figure that out, start the recovery process, and you will be well on your way to achieving and maintaining a healthy weight for life.

Where Do I Start?

~ · ~ · ~ ~ · ~ · ~ · ~

Although I have given you many examples, *probably too many*, from my own life, I know you must be wondering, "Where do *I* start?" How do *I* change my life and habits so *I* can lose weight and keep it off once and for all? The answer is actually surprisingly simple... I think you should start off by spending some quiet time alone, it can be as little as fifteen minutes or as long as you need, to come up with a list of goals that you would like to achieve where your body and health are concerned. The goals you set should be *realistic* and *measurable*. As an example, "I would like to be a size 8, 10, 12, or 14 (*whatever* **your** *picture is*) by a specific date in the future," or "I would like to lower my blood pressure or cholesterol reading by a certain amount by a certain date" (*your doctor may need to help you decide this one*). My lists usually include multiple goals such as getting to a specific weight, being able to wear a certain size or outfit, being able to run a mile without stopping, etc.

Regardless of what winds up on your list, it should all be approached with the following statement, "*What Can I Do Today?*" The answer to your long-term success lies in what you can commit to each day—literally taking each endeavor one day at a time. Any other way is too overwhelming. For this reason, I have included a worksheet at the end of this chapter to help you identify specific things you can do today where *your* eating, physical activity, and health are concerned. In every area of your life you must remember that pursuing and achieving goals always starts with first steps, sometimes baby ones, when it comes to losing weight, such as:

- *What can I do to eat a healthier breakfast?*
- *Could I walk to get lunch instead of driving?*
- *Can I skip the soda at lunch and drink water instead?*
- *How about eating fruit or soup with a sandwich instead of chips or fries for lunch?*
- *What if I ate more vegetables at dinner and less bread?*
- *What about walking around the block or driving to a park/track and just walking or jogging around it once after dinner?*

No pressure, *just focus on what you can do today without freaking out*. I know there may be things you cannot, or may not be ready to do, so **only focus on what you can do RIGHT NOW**. Remember in my first wake-up call how I started off with small steps (*i.e., replacing regular bread with low-calorie bread, whole milk with 1 percent milk and sodas with water*)? Well, over time those small steps helped me to reach the goals that had once seemed unreachable. I know that what I have learned may not be the 100 percent answer for everyone, but I am sure that you have heard something that can help you think of areas/habits that you should change or at least tweak. So start looking at your life, and come up with ideas on how you can make healthier, wiser choices that you can live with for a lifetime. Start small, keep it simple, and go slow…

Resist the Temptation

I believe most diets and weight loss programs fail us because they try to make us do too much too soon. They unrealistically expect dieters to change habits overnight that may have taken a lifetime to develop. You are expected to go from not eating right and not exercising to being a poster child for health and fitness—*not eating many of the foods you like and being a regular at the gym*. During the first few days it usually feels really good, and we go in with the best intentions as we declare, "*This time will be different! I am finally going to lose the weight!*"Believe me, I know because I have been at this point many times before. However, after having been there and done that, I know that the average person, *who does not have a genuine love for working out*, will not continue to wake up at 5:00 in the morning to work out at the gym for an hour five or six times a week! I know I could never keep this up unless my life literally depended on it or if someone were paying me millions of dollars to do it!

In addition to imposing unrealistic workout goals, some would also then have us cut out white flour, sugar, starches, dairy, and fried foods at the same time. I believe this is way too much to get used to all at once, and it would send most of us back to the couch with a bag of chips or cookies feeling like a failure within a week! This is not only unfortunate, but, in my opinion, it is unnecessary. I think trying to change too much at once in your eating and exercise habits is one of the main contributors to the yo-yo dieting cycle. *You start one plan—you can't stick with it, you give up, you lick your wounds for a bit, and then you look for the next "new thing."* I also think this explains why there is always such buzz when a new diet book is released, regardless of how nonsensical it may seem. Instead of another diet, I think many of us are really searching for a program or regimen that can be easily incorporated into our everyday lives—one that allows us to live normally in this culture, eating the foods we enjoy like everyone else. *Right?*

I don't know why so many weight loss/fitness/health professionals and writers take such an all-or-nothing approach where weight loss and healthy eating are concerned, especially when I know such extremes are not required. If they were, I would be as big as a house! I really don't believe that your life has to radically change overnight in order for you to reach your weight loss goals. *I just don't.* In fact, even as I think about it, a saying comes to mind that talks about the race not always going to the swift or fast, but to those that take it slow and steady (paraphrasing of course). Remember the race between the hare and the tortoise? In case you forgot, the tortoise won even though he was obviously slower. That is what comes to mind when I think about the process of losing weight and keeping it off, especially during times when I see women running by me as I am out walking or who are at the gym for an hour or more while I am walking in my neighborhood or on my treadmill watching TV. Some of them are slimmer and in better shape than I am, but a good number of them are not. Running and/or working out at the gym may be right for them, but it is not necessarily right for me. I can lose weight and keep it off just by walking consistently.

I believe the secret to my success where my weight loss goals are concerned is doing what is right/works for me, and that is what I am encouraging you to do. Trust me, you will need to make a lot of little changes here and there (*in later chapters I will give you suggestions and tips to help you with this*) that you can live with over time in order to successfully lose and keep off a significant amount of weight. However, no matter what path you choose to reach your goals, I urge you to resist the temptation to make it an all-or-nothing proposition, and just focus on doing what you can do today. Don't spend too much time worrying about all of the things you are not doing or giving up. That will only stress you out more, *making you want to eat even more and do even less*. For this reason, I strongly urge you to just turn all of your attention to what you *CAN DO NOW*, and just *DO IT*!

The Most Trivialized Addiction

As you start on your path to losing weight and keeping it off, taking *one step at a time*, I do realize that some may have it harder than others. For those who abuse/have abused food (i.e., prone to uncontrollable or emotional eating, etc.), you may have a battle similar to someone who struggles with alcohol or drugs in the sense that it is a day-by-day battle that you never conquer—*you just keep taking it one step at a time for the rest of your life so you don't fall back into old destructive patterns*. While I am not necessarily comparing the hardship of a person with a weight problem to that of someone with a drug or alcohol addiction, I do believe that food can be our drug of choice. *It is mine*. When I am upset, tired, cranky, or overwhelmed there is nothing more I would love to do than to get in my bed with a pack of *Keebler Fudge Covered Graham Crackers*, the same way some might feel about needing a drink, and I don't think that will *ever* change. However, most of the time I resist the urge, and with each day of doing the right thing, it becomes easier to resist these types of impulses. However, it is a daily struggle, which makes me think that it is a form of addiction.

The same impulses and voids in your life that might lead you to drugs or alcohol can also lead you to overeat, but trying to beat a food addiction can sometimes be even harder. One of the reasons I say this is because at least programs that help you deal with drug or alcohol addictions tell you to never have the addictive item again—*alcoholics should never drink alcohol, cocaine addicts should never use cocaine, etc*. However, for those of us who struggle with food, you can't just say, don't have any more food. The very thing you are addicted to is the thing that you have to have every day of your life to live and be healthy. Just like a popular fast food chain says, "*You Gotta Eat!*," and it's true, for the most part, you have got to eat EVERY single day… Buying food, making choices, preparing it for yourself and others, smelling it, handling it and deciding when and how much to eat *over and over again*. I think on some levels this is like an alcoholic working in a bar, seven days a week, twenty-four hours a day because every day, everywhere you go you are faced with your biggest temptation. So for this reason, I think food addictions can be a little harder to deal with, but again, I would never want to diminish the struggle that people face with drug/alcohol addictions. Either way, I think you get my point.

So as you deal with possible food addictions and/or eating habits that led you to where you are today, the next few chapters will help you to:

- Assess Where You Are Today and Make a Commitment to Change;
- Identify What's *Eating* You;
- Relax & Rethink Your Life;
- Request & Receive Help;
- Rev Up & Revolutionize Your Activity; and
- Redefine & Reshape Your Eating Habits.

No More Shortcuts

Losing weight and keeping it off does not have to be complicated. In fact, the more complicated we make it, the more elusive our weight loss goals may be. If you are going to stick with a plan for the long term and be successful, you cannot be so focused on *have to's* or *can'ts*. For example, I *have to* eat foods from a certain company or program (e.g., *Jenny Craig, Weight Watchers, Nutrisystem*, etc.), I *can't* eat dairy products, or I *can't have* more than a certain number of calories a day. This is such a legalistic approach to life and eating, especially as you try to implement it while living in the real world. This type of thinking often leads to you being even more frustrated and disappointed in the end, looking for yet another diet plan to follow.

Let's be honest, you need a plan that is reasonable and medically sound enough for you to continue on it for a lifetime. *This is the overall goal.* So let's decide right now—NO MORE SHORTCUTS! It's all about our health and what we can commit to for a lifetime. I say this to prepare you for the simple fact that losing weight and keeping it off forever is a proposition that takes time and patience. So that means **no diet pills, no meal replacements** *unless prescribed by a doctor,* **no low-calorie diets, no meal skipping, no long-term fasting** *unless for religious or medical purposes,* **no purging, no laxatives/diuretics**, and **no surgery** *unless it is medically necessary.* We have to stop looking for a *miracle* that will make the weight go away. I will admit that over the years I have bought products claiming to do just that. Did they work? *Of course not.* **There are no miracle cures for weight loss.** The only miracle is that we have the power to change our weight and our lives if we want. We just have to be realistic about what we are prepared to do…

Can you really eat *Jenny Craig's* food for a lifetime, and with the cost, would you even want to? Can you live on 1,500 calories a day for the rest of your life? Will you go to the gym every morning at 5:30 a.m. for the long term? Do you want your stomach permanently reduced to a size where you can no longer eat normal-sized meals? *I don't think so.* This is why I recommend a slow process that involves gradual changes—cutting out foods that you won't miss here and there, replacing not-so-healthy choices with healthier ones and moving however you like, every chance you get. Weight is not gained overnight, it happens over time. As a result, it will be lost over time as well…

So here's to your brand new start, and to cheer you on, I have included a few do's and don'ts for you to remember:

Do's

✓ Get a physical before starting this, or any other, weight loss regimen, and don't stop there; schedule other medical appointments too (e.g., mammograms, teeth cleaning, etc.). An ounce of prevention is really worth a pound of cure!

✓ Treat your weight loss/maintenance goal as a lifelong endeavor, so falling off the wagon temporarily does not matter because *you are in this for the long term, not as a quick fix.*

✓ Work to incorporate healthy eating habits and exercise opportunities that you can live with and enjoy in your daily routine.

✓ Remove the word "diet" from your vocabulary.

✓ Focus on your health and quality of life.

✓ Take time out for you, and get in touch with struggles/stress you may not be dealing with.

✓ Be good to yourself as well as to those around you.

✓ Spend time cultivating hobbies and pursuing passions.

✓ Realize your value/worth without regard to your weight—*you are not your weight*, so do not let anyone define you by it. Commit to living the life you want to live **before** you start trying to lose weight.

✓ Adopt a *can-do* attitude. Focus on what you *can* do, not what you *can't* do, and then do it!

Don'ts

✓ Don't waste any time thinking about all the times you may have failed in the past as you tried to lose weight.

✓ Don't give any merit to negative or hurtful things that anyone has said to put you down regarding your weight or any other area of your life. **You are not defined by your past, mistakes, or shortcomings.**

✓ Don't spend time worrying about what you are going to eat beyond the current meal.

✓ Don't compare your body or progress to other people (*this is the one I have to work on*).

✓ Do not sit around bored or feeling sorry for yourself—if you feel you don't have a life, go out and create one! If you can't think of anything, volunteer to help others until you can!

✓ Don't let anyone's perception of you hold you back.

✓ Don't ever give up on yourself or any other goal you set for yourself. You are worth second, third, and fourth chances—however many you may need. Just keep getting back up, and make whatever you want happen in your life.

✓ Don't ever believe that you can't get your weight under control because YOU CAN!!!!!!!!!!!!!!

So this is where you start, *WITH YOU*—*who you are, what you want and what you are prepared to do today to get to where you want to be in the future*. Sounds simple, huh? Unfortunately, it is not as simple as we'd like. However, I think the next few sections should make things a little easier, but on your way there I suggest you spend some time filling out the sheet on the next page. It is a great exercise to help you brainstorm and see what ideas you can come up with that you are willing to do *today* to help you reach your goals. I bet you will come up with something really good! So go ahead and write it down. Then we can move on to the juicy, life-changing sections ahead.

WHAT CAN I DO TODAY
TO REACH MY WEIGHT LOSS GOAL?

What / When / How / Where I Eat...
(Are there changes, substitutions, reductions, or deletions that I can make with the following meals? Are there foods / drinks / condiments I can live without?)

- **Breakfast** _____

- **Mid-morning Snack** _____

- **Lunch** _____

- **Afternoon Snack(s)** _____

- **Dinner** _____

- **Evening Snack(s)** _____

Incorporating More Activity Into My Routine...
(What can I start doing? What can I do differently? What else can I do?)

- **Morning Routine** _____

- **At Work** _____

- **During Lunch** _____

- **After Work / Dinner** _____

Improving My Environment at Home and Work...
(How can I make my environment more conducive to healthy eating and being active?)

_____

_____

_____

~

Assess Where You Are &
Make A Commitment
To Change...
~ . ~ . ~ ~ . ~ . ~ . ~

I would like to start this chapter off by saying that I believe the size you are now is a reflection of the person you were *before* you made the decision to change your life—*not of who you are now or who you will become in the future*. I think this is a very important point to make because you must start seeing yourself as the person you are "now"—the *one you have decided to be*, and start thinking like *that* new person, instead of like the person you once *were*. One of the reasons many of us fail to make long-term changes where our bodies are concerned is *because we often continue thinking like the person we used to be. As a result, we repeat the same eating and behavior patterns that led us to be overweight in the first place.*

So why not start the ball rolling by taking a good, long look in the mirror to assess where you are with your weight as a result of the person that you *"were."* Get the scale out, and see where you *really* are. If you can, also go to the doctor to get your blood pressure, cholesterol and blood sugar readings. In fact, get all the information you can regarding your current condition. Were you shocked by what you found out? If so, that's OK, but don't let it get you down. Feel free to cry if you'd like. *Feel* whatever you are feeling, it is a part of the process. *This is your wake-up call.* You have heard about mine, *but this one is yours.* It is your turn to say, *"I don't wanna go out like this. This is not who I am. This is not how I envisioned my life! I am finally going to transform myself into the person that I really am!"*

Where Am I Really?

On our own, I know it can be hard to objectively determine where we really are in terms of how much weight we need to lose to be healthy. "Looking good" in our clothes is certainly not a true indicator. This is where doctors and organizations such as *The U.S. Department of Health and Human Services* and the *National Institutes of Health* come in. These organizations have Web sites that can help us determine our body mass index (BMI), a measure of body fat based on height and weight that applies to both adult men and women. The BMI is a reliable indicator of total body fat, which is related to the risk of disease and death. Check out http://win.niddk.nih.gov to see the following BMI table:

Body Mass Index Table

To calculate your BMI, find your height in the left-hand column, and move across to find your weight. The number at the top of the column where your height and weight meet is your BMI.

BMI	19	20	21	22	23	24	25	26	27	28	29	30	31	32	33	34	35	36	37	38	39	40
Height (inches)								Body Weight (pounds)														
58	91	96	100	105	110	115	119	124	129	134	138	143	148	153	158	162	167	172	177	181	186	191
59	94	99	104	109	114	119	124	128	133	138	143	148	153	158	163	168	173	178	183	188	193	198
60	97	102	107	112	118	123	128	133	138	143	148	153	158	163	168	174	179	184	189	194	199	204
61	100	106	111	116	122	127	132	137	143	148	153	158	164	169	174	180	185	190	195	201	206	211
62	104	109	115	120	126	131	136	142	147	153	158	164	169	175	180	186	191	196	202	207	213	218
63	107	113	118	124	130	135	141	146	152	158	163	169	175	180	186	191	197	203	208	214	220	225
64	110	116	122	128	134	140	145	151	157	163	169	174	180	186	192	197	204	209	215	221	227	232
65	114	120	126	132	138	144	150	156	162	168	174	180	186	192	198	204	210	216	222	228	234	240
66	118	124	130	136	142	148	155	161	167	173	179	186	192	198	204	210	216	223	229	235	241	247
67	121	127	134	140	146	153	159	166	172	178	185	191	198	204	211	217	223	230	236	242	249	255
68	125	131	138	144	151	158	164	171	177	184	190	197	203	210	216	223	230	236	243	249	256	262
69	128	135	142	149	155	162	169	176	182	189	196	203	209	216	223	230	236	243	250	257	263	270
70	132	139	146	153	160	167	174	181	188	195	202	209	216	222	229	236	243	250	257	264	271	278
71	136	143	150	157	165	172	179	186	193	200	208	215	222	229	236	243	250	257	265	272	279	286
72	140	147	154	162	169	177	184	191	199	206	213	221	228	235	242	250	258	265	272	279	287	294
73	144	151	159	166	174	182	189	197	204	212	219	227	235	242	250	257	265	272	280	288	295	302
74	148	155	163	171	179	186	194	202	210	218	225	233	241	249	256	264	272	280	287	295	303	311
75	152	160	168	176	184	192	200	208	216	224	232	240	248	256	264	272	279	287	295	303	311	319
76	156	164	172	180	189	197	205	213	221	230	238	246	254	263	271	279	287	295	304	312	320	328

Source: Clinical Guidelines on Identification, Evaluation, and Treatment of Overweight and Obesity in Adults, NHLBI, September 1998

BMI Categories:

- Underweight = <18.5
- Normal weight = 18.5-24.9
- Overweight = 25-29.9
- Obesity = BMI of 30 or greater

I already know what many of you may be thinking… How can some arbitrary indicator tell me whether I am at a healthy weight, overweight, or obese just based on my height, especially when *the makers of the chart have never seen me, don't know my bone structure, body type, etc.?* To a certain extent, you are right because I am sure it cannot accurately assess all cases. This is why I think you should view your BMI reading as a guideline that can point out dangerous weights for your height or acceptable ranges that you should try to stay within. With that said, proponents of BMI charts/readings have also pointed out a few of the limitations that should be considered as individuals use them to determine their weight loss goals:

- Readings may **overestimate** body fat in athletes and others who have a muscular build.
- Readings may **underestimate** body fat in older people and those who have lost muscle mass.

Even with these caveats, I still think your BMI is a very useful indicator for determining the healthiest weight for you to reach *and* maintain. When you visit your doctor, be sure to take this information with you so you can have a discussion about what this reading means to you/your health and where you need to be based on his or her professional opinion *and* your medical history. I think this is one of the best ways for you to determine your goal weight.

Don't Do It!

I know this section can be scary and intimidating for those of you whose readings fall into the obese category (*a BMI greater than/equal to 30*) or the overweight category (*a BMI of 25 to 29.9*). However, I don't want you to panic or mentally check out, and move on to the next chapter or worse, put the book down. *Please, don't do it!* Knowledge is power. So now that you know what you are up against, *you have the power to do something about it!* You can turn this around, so do not blow it off. This is the time to use your power to acknowledge what you know, and ***take action!*** The key is to think and act in small steps so you don't become overwhelmed. That is a theme you will find throughout this book because small, consistent steps are the best way to ensure long-term success in almost any endeavor. Did you know that even a small weight loss (*just 10 percent of your current weight*) could help lower the risk of your developing diseases associated with obesity (*e.g., high blood cholesterol, type 2 diabetes, heart disease, stroke, certain cancers, etc.*)? Well, you won't get the chance to change things if you don't acknowledge where you are and move forward. *So like Nike says, "Just Do It!"*

Take the Information & Move Forward

Now that you know your BMI, hopefully you have gone or will go to the doctor to get all of your vitals (e.g., blood pressure, cholesterol reading, blood sugar level, etc.), and you **are ready to do what's required to get healthy.** If you haven't, I want to take one more opportunity to convince you to do it... *I know* everyone's body, height, and metabolism are different... I *know* it can be tempting to say being overweight/obese is OK if we look good in our clothes, or if we are smaller than some of our colleagues, friends, or family members. Yeah, yeah, yeah... Well, regardless of our height, build, *or* how sexy we are, we should all have the same goal—*to get to the healthiest weight we can*. I say this because our hearts, blood vessels, joints, and tendons don't care how good we *think* we look in our clothes or how sexy we *think* we are. If you think I am wrong, think of how many beautiful, *sexy* people we know with type 2 diabetes, high cholesterol, hypertension, etc. We can fool people, but we can't fool our bodies (e.g., major systems, organs, etc.), which *do* care and *are* impacted by how much we weigh. As a result, I urge you to make it a priority to determine where you are weight- and health-wise, and figure out where you need to be/how much weight you want to lose as soon as possible. Like I said, talk to your doctor if you need help or guidance. *That's what doctors are there for, right?*

Once you know where you are *and* where you want to go in terms of your weight, *and* you are truly committed to getting there, there is another critical step you must take... You must accept the fact that *the weight you are trying to lose was not gained overnight, and it will not be lost overnight.* So don't lose hope or get discouraged just as you are getting started. You have to remember that you are in this for the long haul. There is a Bible scripture that speaks to this, "*... let us not be weary in well doing: for in due season we shall reap, if we faint not*" (Galatians 6:9). Translation: If we keep doing the right things (*i.e., dealing with emotional issues/stress, making better food choices, being more active, etc.*) without giving up, we will be rewarded (*i.e., weight loss, improved health, etc.*). Holding on to this thought is absolutely critical to keeping your morale up and ensuring your long-term success. So with that out of the way, let me say that *this is your time to really make it happen!* Believe me, ***you can do it!*** You just have to *decide* that this time you *really, really* want it, and then go ahead and commit yourself to doing it—*one step at a time, one day at a time*. No matter how many times you have to pick yourself up and try it again... **Just keep moving forward.** It is just that simple (*well, maybe not simple, but you know what I mean*).

What's *Eating* You?
~ · ~ · ~ ~ · ~ · ~ · ~

"You will not cry! OK, *Carolyn, let's try to keep it together. You are not going to cry in front of all of these people! I am not going to cry! I will not cry! Oh my goodness, I am crying.* OK, *not another tear. Please, Lord, help me get myself together. Oh, Lord, why am I crying? I thought I was so over this... Why am I not over this?????"* These are just a few of the thoughts that were racing through my mind on Sunday, September 24, 2006, during my sister-in-law's CD release celebration. She is an up-and-coming gospel artist, and I was enjoying the songs she was performing from her CD until she sang the one called *"A Father's Love."* It was such a beautiful song, and everyone else was enjoying it and celebrating. However, this song surprisingly cut me to the core in a profoundly sad way, and a lifetime of tears that had not been shed threatened to pour any minute...

Even though my estranged father died a month before this event, without us ever reconciling, I *thought* I was OK. I don't recall feeling sad or mournful. I didn't hate him. I didn't feel particularly angry or bitter at that point. *In fact, I don't recall feeling anything.* My father lived a very tragic, selfish life where, for whatever reasons, he seemed incapable of giving of himself. I think the way he was raised had a great deal to do with that. Be that as it may, he never rose above it, and in a life of sixty plus years, there was no one at the end who had anything good to say about him... Sadly enough, the only good thing I could think of was that he was my father, and like it or not, without him, I wouldn't be here. Also, as my son pointed out, there are a few close cousins that we wouldn't have otherwise.

That's it. That was his memorial and what I walked away with. However, that obviously was not enough closure for me. Otherwise, why were the thoughts I had during my sister-in-law's CD release party enough to make me want to cry hysterically? I don't think I was sad or mourning my father because I never really knew him, and he was never really a part of my life. So maybe I was mourning what I never had and *never would have—A Father's Love.* Something that even today I realize I missed. Before his death there was hope, but now that chapter of my life was forever closed... Death brought such finality. *Surprisingly, the closing of that door helped me understand a lot about my past behavior and eating habits...*

A Flash Back in Time

There was a time when it literally felt like I was eating from the time I woke up until the time I fell asleep. I remember waking up with a half-eaten, smashed *Little Debbie Swiss Cake Roll* under my pillow. ***I WAS ALWAYS EATING***, and much of it was done unconsciously. As a teenager and during my early twenties I spent quite a bit of time overeating (*not saying that I never occasionally overeat now because there are times that I do*), and I thought it was just because I loved to eat candy bars and cookies. *It wasn't.* I know now it was about a lot more than that. However, you usually don't have this type of clarity until you are looking back in hindsight. You know the saying, *hindsight really is 20-20.*

I can remember spending weekends with one of my "slim" cousins as a teenager, and I would ask her to stop at a convenience store on the way to her house because I wanted to get *something*. When I would ask her if she wanted *something*, she usually said no and kinda looked at me like I was crazy as I bought my sixteen-ounce soda and high-fat/high-sugar snack. She may not have *needed* a snack at the time, but I literally *needed* one. It almost felt like I was experiencing a mild form of withdrawal, as it had been a few hours since we had last eaten (it could have been as few as one), but I couldn't wait for my next *fix*. I just couldn't go any longer, and something inside of me was saying, "*You have got to eat something now!*" Hunger never entered the equation because I knew I was not hungry, but *something* kept driving me to eat. I just couldn't help myself, and I didn't know it then, but food was my drug of choice, and I reached for it any time I felt anxious or was *feeling something I didn't want to feel*. Something was "eating me," but I just didn't know what.

During those weekends at my cousin's house, I literally could not wait to go back to the solace of my own home, where I could eat *what* I wanted, *when* I wanted. At home, no one could witness me eating three or four ice cream sandwiches back-to-back, while drinking glass after glass of *Kool-Aid*, ice tea, or soda, as I sat on the sofa watching TV. Snacking on junk-food was my habit, my addiction… It was a temporary and *ineffective* fix for what ailed me, but in the absence of anything better, I continued the cycle. Out of desperation, I remember trying over-the-counter diet pills in college, hoping I would lose weight and stop overeating. However, I never lost a pound because I would forget that I had taken the doggone pills and grab food out of habit just as I did before taking them. *What was wrong with me that diet pills and their twelve-hour release formula could not cure????* I didn't know then, but I do now…

What Was Eating Me?

So what was wrong me? What was *eating me* during my times of massive overeating? I didn't know it back then, but the death of my father forced me to recall many of the feelings I suppressed as a child and as a young woman. After having children I became more in touch with my feelings, and I have been working through them ever since. I really didn't know all of the *stuff* I was mad about *below the surface* until I started writing this book. During the process, I noticed the recurring theme seems to be *my father, my family,* and *a lack of connection with almost all of them, as well as isolation.*

For many years, I did not feel close to hardly any member of my family—*not my father, mother, cousins, grandparents, aunts, or uncles.* In fact, I can only remember a few family members, *if any,* ever hugging me or saying they loved me or were proud of me. As a result, I began to view family as a complete and utter waste of time. Even from an ancestral perspective, I only heard negative stories, so I didn't care to hear or learn more. I can't even remember the names of my great-grandparents. Everyone in my family was basically written off in my mind, and I built an almost-impenetrable wall around myself and decided that none of them could be trusted. At that time I felt, "*None of you are rooting for me, so I refuse to be emotionally available to any of you, and you will never, ever get another chance.*"

Before I realized it, this attitude of distrust and disconnection began to extend to everyone I came in contact with, *even my husband...* In fact, he had a major battle to fight just to get me past the point where every question I asked was not a third-degree interrogation. Finally, he told me if I didn't start trusting someone, I would wind up alone. Because I loved him, and he had proven himself to be worthy of my trust, I allowed him access to my self-imposed fortress and later our kids, but other people could forget about it! This lack of connection even affects me today, as I often wonder why I have not maintained friendships from the past. I can't point the finger at other people, it is obviously me...

Sure I am outgoing, I talk and joke a lot, and I *superficially* know a lot of people, but I have very few close emotional connections with family and non-family other than my husband and children. I have only one cousin that I am in contact with on a regular basis, as well as my mom and my great-aunt. There is only one friend from high school that I may talk to every few years and only one friend from college I have talked to about three times since graduating. I have made some close friends since leaving college, *but very few*. So my life before the husband and kids was pretty lonely, and even today I struggle to interact with people on a close and personal level, which makes me a loner and socially inept in some ways...

My Emotional Laundry List

It is funny that I can see all of this so clearly now, but I couldn't see the extent of my pain back then. I didn't really, *really* find out the depth, breadth and weight of it until the death of my father, which forced me to recall many of the feelings I suppressed as a child and a young woman. *I remember feeling sad. I remember feeling lonely, isolated and disconnected. I also remember being inexplicably angry*, but I never knew why, and because my mother was the only one around, most of it was directed at her. *I remember being ashamed of myself and my circumstances.* I was a mess of jumbled up feelings and angst, but they all seemed to be expressed as anger. I never could pinpoint the exact feelings I felt then, but anger and sarcasm were my companions. Sometimes they still are, but as I said I have been working through all of this suppressed garbage for years. However, I *finally* know what I was suppressing, *what was eating me* all of those years, and here it is:

- I was deeply hurt by the fact that I never heard from my father on my birthday, holidays, graduations, etc. He never even called after the fact to apologize or make up for it. It was as if either he forgot these days/events existed, or *he forgot I existed*. There were no gifts, no cards, no visits or long periods of time spent together and **no** good memories to speak of. I can't even begin to explain how much that hurt, and how that hurt still lingers to this day. This was painfully obvious as I struggled to listen to the song my sister-in-law sang about a father's love.

  Another aspect that added to this pain was being constantly told that my father was no good and being able to *see* qualities and actions that supported those assessments for myself. There was no room to be delusional or naive where his character was concerned. Be that as it may, I still recall longing to see him *even though he lived less than ten miles from us*. I remember bugging my mom about watching the Christmas parade that runs between Augusta, Georgia and North Augusta, South Carolina (the cities are separated by a bridge) on the South Carolina side because someone mentioned seeing my father there once. I would have never admitted it then, but I was just hoping to catch a glimpse of him. Maybe he would see me and suddenly remember he had a daughter that needed him. Maybe seeing me would jog his memory, and maybe, *just maybe*, he would feel guilty or sorry that he left me. Maybe we would have one of those emotional moments like you see on television, and he would say he was sorry, and we could pick up where we left off… Well, we never got to watch the parade on that side of the bridge because the people that took us always watched it from the Georgia side, and I could never bring myself to admit to my mom why this was so important to me. So the father-daughter reunion never happened, and I eventually stopped asking, but for years this type of *stuff* ate at me, and the very thought of it could make me cry. *Even today, it could if I let it…*

- Not having a father was bad enough, but I also grew up without brothers or sisters (*my father had two sons with another woman while he was married to my mother, but I never knew them*). I met and talked to one of them for the first time after I graduated college, but unfortunately *we were just strangers with the same father...* I had no one with a shared history, and I really missed not having that... I would have loved to talk to someone who was dealing with the same issues/circumstances that I was. Someone else who understood where I was coming from without me having to explain everything... I just wanted to be able to say to a brother, sister or close relative something that most people take for granted, *"Remember that time* that we did *blah* or went *blah?"* Then you laugh or cry about the stories that made up your childhood, and you share those stories with your children. I think this gives a person a sense of family ties or history, which unfortunately I never felt/had until I got married.

- Added on to the "father" issues, was one of the most hurtful things I can recall from my past. It was a time when my father's mother, who I used to think I loved more than anyone else in the world, became angry with me. *I think it was because I would not eat the meatloaf she had me make, which was loaded with breadcrumbs, onions and bell peppers — Yuck!* She had the nerve to tell me, *"You are going to be no good, just like your ole daddy."* She then went on to tell me how my cousin (the *"slim"* one), who was a few months older than me, was more ladylike and implied she was a better person. Here I was a good student, *doing the best I could without her son's support*, and more importantly, I loved her. I even spent two boring weeks helping her that summer, *and this was the thanks I got?* Another summer almost over, and the start of *another* school year where I would not be able to afford to buy school clothes like many of the kids at my school had (I so desperately wanted the preppy clothes I saw in *Seventeen* magazine that year) because *her* son couldn't keep a job and wouldn't help support me!

I was only fourteen, but that moment was life-defining for me. I was emotionally done with **everyone** in my family, especially my grandmother and my father. *Even the people who may not have actually done anything to me...* I did not respond to what she said, but the way I looked at her let her see the seriousness of what she had said, and that it could never be undone. Almost prophetically she asked as I left to go home, *"I guess I won't be seeing you anymore?"* I immediately said, *"No."* She died a few months later, and my mother tried to break the news in the most delicate way possible given my *past* closeness with my grandmother. I remember I was in my room reading at the time, and after she told me, I just said, "*That's too bad.*" Then I went back to reading my book. I never cried. I never even recall feeling sad or anything other than a passing thought of, "*Oh well.*"

I didn't want to go to her funeral, and my mother didn't make me. Given the great love I had for this woman, it is amazing how quickly I cut her off. I am sad now that I cannot even remember what she looked like, even though I have tried over the past few years to see her face in my mind. In hindsight, I do remember her acting erratically during that last visit, so I am sure complications from diabetes may have been to blame for some of her outburst. I was just too angry to see that until now... However, from that moment on, I began cutting people off mentally and emotionally if they even came close to hurting me. It has become an automatic defense response, which can make me very touchy, unforgiving and isolated...

• Although the "slim" cousin I mentioned earlier reached out to me when I was a teenager, I was very distrustful of my father's side of the family because I had not spent time with them. I guess I thought they only cared about me because I resembled my cousin (just heavier and shorter). Also, I am sure I was embarrassed because some people on that side didn't know who I was or how I was related to them. To get them to know, I had to say that I was *his* daughter, which brought a whole lot of baggage and embarrassment with it because they either knew his history *or* didn't know him at all.

Even at a family reunion recently, I couldn't bring myself to mention his name when I was trying to get a distant cousin to know who I was. *I didn't want his history to be my history.* I finally mentioned my mother's name, and fortunately that was enough, but for a moment I was very uncomfortable, and I *became that embarrassed little girl again.* This was enough to make me realize that I am *still* embarrassed today, and I have never felt like an official member of that family, and in many ways I don't think I ever will... As an adult, I can live with that, but as a child that was a hard and bitter pill to swallow, especially since I am not close to anyone on my mother's side of the family either. So, to me, it *really* felt like no one cared, especially during the times when my mom and I weren't close.

- I was also painfully conflicted and ashamed regarding the molestation that happened when I was nine. There was guilt, confusion and a myriad of other emotions. However, instead of being mad at the molester, *I was mad at my mother.* I see how irrational that is now, but back then, it just widened the chasm that kept my mother and me from being close over the years. Things did not really improve until I told her about *it* and a lot of other things I was unhappy about growing up. This was around the time I turned forty. Until this point, my anger prevented us from having a good relationship. Fortunately we are on a better footing and have a very healthy relationship now, but for many years, this craziness ate away at me.

- I am sad to say there is even more... For years I looked to my mother, father and extended family for validation of my worth as a person. I think I wanted someone to say, *"Good Job," "We are proud of you," "You can become anything you want to become," "We are behind you," "You are destined for great things,"*– basically all of the usual good things kids want/need to hear. When I did not hear these things from them, but heard a lot of negative, discouraging comments instead, to say I was *angry* was an understatement. Until I met my husband in college, I had thoughts of moving to Europe and never seeing any of them again! Obviously this is what I was thinking at eighteen and nineteen. Although I only moved to Virginia, I still remained very angry with them. I know now that I was looking for confirmation from *them* that I was okay and that I could do the things that I believed I could do, and when they didn't give it, I was hurt. I didn't know it then, but *the validation I sought comes from within...*

- I tell you, the bitterness and rot in my heart from the past with the whole family thing has really taken its toll on me. It has been so hard moving past the bad feelings towards my family, especially since I have never confronted anyone or blown up at anyone other than my mother about my feelings. Most of this has been suppressed until now... The only time I came close to wanting to let everyone *have it* was during one of the angriest moments of my life. Surprisingly, this was a few days before my wedding, *one of the happiest days of my life*— tying with the birth of my children. However, I felt like a hissing rattle snake poised to strike as people were telling me that I needed someone to walk down the aisle with me. I remember feeling tremendous rage as my mom suggested that one of my uncles/her brother give me away. I am sure she wanted my wedding experience to be as nice as possible, but I would not hear of it because I could not remember one encouraging word this person had ever said to me. Also, I wanted my wedding to be touching like the ones you see in movies (think *Father of the Bride* or *My Big Fat Greek Wedding* where someone who really loves you walks you down the aisle).

Unfortunately there was no male relative that was ever there for me when I really needed someone, and in my bitterness, I was thinking I certainly didn't need any of them now! This whole thought process led me to get even angrier about my dad, or lack thereof, and I decided that I was going to walk down the aisle alone! I felt if I had walked alone this far, with only God to fall back on, then that was how I would walk down the aisle! However, after being harassed a bit by people involved in the wedding, I did finally decide to walk down the aisle with my husband's uncle. *I didn't know him very well, but at least I liked him.* Be that as it may, it still hurt me that my special day was tainted by bitterness from my past, and that *I was given away by someone who I barely knew, and who barely knew me...*

Am I a big mess of emotional issues or what? That sure is a lot of baggage to be carried around by one person, and these are just a few of the big ticket issues! It is funny that as I write this, I remember that my husband gave me the nickname *"Quick"* because he said I am quick to get mad, but also quick to cool down. However, he has jokingly asked me over the years, *"Why are you so mad all the time?"* Usually I would joke back and tell him about the pointless thing(s) that I might have been mad about at the time, but I was not fully aware of all of the *stuff* I was *really* mad about *below the surface* until I started writing this book. To be able to successfully articulate what has been eating me over the last thirty plus years, without spending thousands of dollars on therapy, is incredible and very cathartic.

Hopefully it won't take you as long to have your breakthrough! I have always heard that the first step to working through and moving beyond a problem is to understand and acknowledge it. As you have heard so far, I have done that at great length, but I must admit that I am still not over all that ails me, and I can't say whether I ever will be completely… There is still residual anger that appears occasionally. So although I have worked through many of my issues, there is still a mountain of hurt/anger that I am processing and releasing. After much prayer and soul searching, I decided to work to let go of the anger and bitterness that used to eat away at me. In fact, one of my daily affirmations is, "***I have let go of all anger and bitterness toward those who have hurt me, and I love them the way God would want me to.***" I think it is helping, but it takes time.

My healing started with the realization that *the people that hurt me did not do it deliberately.* Their behavior was based on what was going on with them at the time and/or their life experiences. ***They didn't mean it personally***, but I took it personally. I was wrong. *It is not all about me. The world does not revolve around me, and I need to get over myself.* This is the tough-love talk I use sometimes when I am talking to myself. So just like that, it was time to let it all go. I can't take any credit because I believe God is healing my heart, as I have been praying for years to be free from the hurt and pain of my past. A part of that process has been to turn my focus outward and to be more concerned about the feelings or difficulties of others and what may have led them to act the way they have. I still have a *long, long* way to go, but I feel a lot more peaceful, and I now try to deal with my problems more directly. The surprising reward is that *the more I do this, the less I need food as a crutch…*

Is Something *Eating* You?

OK, now you know in great detail what has been eating me (*and still does occasionally*) and how I am handling it, but what about you? Do you have some issue(s) that you are wrestling with? *Is there something eating you???* Only you know for sure… As you think about it, keep in mind that *it can take many years to know all that eats you (I know it has for me).* However, the purpose of this exercise is to get you to start the soul-searching process and see what issues/reasons you can come up with that could be related (*directly or indirectly*) to your eating habits. *So don't take it lightly.* To facilitate your thought process, feel free to write down thoughts as they come to you (*now or later on in the book*):

_____

_____

_____

_____

_____

_____

_____

One of the reasons I decided to include this chapter is because I see so many of us obsessing about *what* we are eating and how many calories/how much fat/how many carbs it has, yet we spend very little time understanding *why* we are eating what we are eating. Well this is the chapter where you uncover what is making you eat so much. Until you identify and find a way to deal with these problems, the excess weight will never go away. It may leave for a time, but it will never stay away for long. I remember hearing Oprah say that she used to think that her weight problem was caused by the fact that she just liked to eat potato chips, but she has since learned better. A revelation like this is the first major step in losing weight and keeping it off—*the acknowledgement that excess weight was not caused by a love of potato chips or any other food.* **That is not the cause of your excess weight either…**   Once you find out the cause, you can be free from the demons of the past, and you can move on to your more enlightened, healthier (*emotionally and physically*) and *slimmer* future.

<u>Moving On</u>
Did you find some areas of hurt and anger that you need to let go of? If you did, you are certainly not alone. Now all you need to do is to acknowledge those areas, work through them, and LET THEM GO once and for all! Make today the day you stop focusing on "why" some event happened or did not happen in your life. Do whatever you need to do to break free from this kind of thinking because it is absolutely toxic. It leads to all sorts of harmful feelings: *self-pity,*

anger, bitterness, depression, etc... As a result, you won't feel good about yourself, which will make you more likely to overeat or turn to food for comfort.

I think a good place to start would be to admit that you don't know why something has/has not happened, and accept the fact that **it does not matter.** It really is what it is, and you have to make the best of it. The "*Why me?*" question must become, "*What will I do next to move forward?*" *How do I prevent an unfortunate event(s) from defining who I am and my future?* As you take your focus off the "*whys,*" the voids you try to fill with food will start to disappear. Focusing on the "*whys*" makes them reappear. I know this for a fact because if I spend too much time focusing on the "*whys*" of my life, I could wind up in bed with a pack of *Keebler Fudge Graham Crackers.* However, I can't let myself go there. My "why" has now become, "*How did God intend me to use this experience to help others?*" I had to face the fact that God allowed me to have the parents, family, and circumstances that I had for a reason... The same goes for you as well. *Would we be the people we are today without the challenges and painful events that happened in our lives?* I don't think so.

There is definitely a lot more good than bad. *However*, if you continue to see a lot more bad than good after much time and prayer, and you have any of the following:

- Thoughts of suicide or violence
- Debilitating depression that you can't work through
- Anorexia, bulimia, or other eating disorders
- Any other emotional issues/problems you just cannot work through on your own

You should speak to your doctor or seek other professional help. Health professionals are here for the purpose of helping us with areas that we can't handle on our own, so there is no shame in asking for help. I think it is important to focus your energy on getting emotionally healthy so that when you do finally lose the weight, it stays off for good!

Chapter 5

R e l a x & R e t h i n k Y o u r L i f e (S t e p 3)

As a child I remember hearing church folk say, *"Let go, and let God,"* and I often wondered, "What are they talking about?" In fact, I used to look at them like they were crazy. I never fully appreciated what that meant, nor did I understand it. *Until now...* OK, OK, I know everyone reading this book may not believe in God or may not have heard the saying, so I will just tell you what it means to me... After long thought, I finally took it to mean that after we have done all we can do, we should turn over our problems, struggles, and hurts to God and let Him help us through them. I don't know about you, but some of my problems have been too big for me to handle on my own, and I needed help getting through them. Do you have any problems or issues that feel too big for you? If so, you are certainly not alone. However, no matter what you are going through, you are going to have to let it go...

This does not mean that you don't have to do the legwork necessary to work through it as I described in the last chapter (e.g., grieving, forgiving someone, accepting things as they are, etc.), but it does mean that you let go of the baggage that is tied to the things you are dealing with. As an example, if you grew up in an environment where people constantly ridiculed you because of your weight or the way you look—your baggage might include desires to get even with them, tell them off, or have nothing ever to do with them again... Maybe you still find yourself replaying scenes/events over and over again in your mind like it just happened yesterday. **Whether you realize it or not, this is mental and emotional baggage, and it weighs on you. It affects your eating, and it can affect your weight.** This type of thinking is not God's best for our lives... It limits us, and keeps us living in the past.

I believe God wants us to live each day to its fullest, not looking back at things we cannot change. I think this is why He gives us special gifts so we can use them to help others while we *get over ourselves* and the experiences that He has helped us make it through. I believe our challenges/troubles have a purpose, and much of it has to do with helping others. Often our pain connects us, and the solutions/answers that we find are not ours alone. *They are meant to be shared.* We were not created to focus on just ourselves and our little problems. This is why when we focus too much on ourselves depression/extreme thoughts can occur. So it is very important that we renew our minds and adjust our focus as needed...

What's Your Focus

A key component in getting your mind right is to turn your focus *outward* instead of inward. This was a lesson I learned inadvertently. As I worked through my personal demons, I found that writing very candid pieces on my life to encourage other women on my Web site helped me deal with my feelings about the past. Surprisingly, the more I did this, the things that were *eating me* slowly became less painful. In fact, I no longer felt the overwhelming desire to get in bed with *Reese's Peanut Butter Cups* or *Little Debbie* snack cakes. I actually found a certain level of fulfillment from encouraging others in the areas I struggled with. This could be the case for you as well. Are there any areas you can think of where you could help others make it through something you are struggling with? *If so, do it.* **Focus outward.**

Guess what happened when I started focusing outward and taking time alone to reflect? **I stopped abusing food.** Also, the cravings to overeat at night began to subside. Now I look forward to doing what I enjoy—getting in bed with my laptop to write, search the Web for information on my latest ideas, read a book or watch a movie/show after a long day of work, cooking dinner, going over homework, working around the house, etc... However, the cool thing is even if my husband is doing something he wants to do or is traveling, I am still OK. I have found purposeful work. My focus is no longer turned solely on me. As a result, I am never bored, and I can comfort and entertain myself *without the help of junk-food or alcohol.*

Find Some "Me" Time

Another way of taking the focus off of *poor little you* is to do something you enjoy on a regular basis. I enjoy reading magazines and self-help books, so when I am not writing/playing around on my laptop, I read. I *aggressively* work to carve out "just for me" time every day, even if it is late at night. During the earlier hours I enjoy spending time with my husband and kids, but as I get to know myself better, I realize I have to have that special time to do what I want to do. One way I do this is by watching movies that I can "veg" out on such as: *Baby Boom* with Diane Keaton, *The Devil Wears Prada* with Anne Hathaway and Meryl Streep, *Something's Gotta Give* again with Diane Keaton, and a crazy movie called *Shirley Valentine* (saved for moments when I *am really* tired/overwhelmed). For some reason movies where women are at a crossroads in their lives help me to mentally escape and go to a place where I can reflect and understand myself better.

Another thing I have learned to do when I am overwhelmed or tired is to let my husband and kids know that my behavior is not a result of what they are doing, but how I am feeling. You know how sometimes you get really, really tired, and you start acting out (*e.g., fussing, nagging, yelling, etc.*)? I get that way sometimes, and I just wanna do what I wanna do, and *sometimes* when that happens, my family allows me to go to a hotel *by myself* or just be home alone for a few hours to write and just *be by myself.* This is absolutely necessary for my mental stability. Maybe it is for you as well... I am more thankful for these gifts of time (e.g., for birthdays, Mother's Day, etc.) than I would be for jewelry or clothes because time alone helps me better understand and handle what ails me.

One of the best things that has come out of my "me" time is the realization that no one can make me happy or solve what ails me—not *my husband, children, friends, or family.* **It is up to me.** Looking to others for happiness, entertainment, or fulfillment leads us down the path of dependency and despair. So I encourage you to spend some time alone (e.g., walking, meditating/in prayer, vegging out, etc.) over the next few months to try to understand yourself better. Purposeful time alone is the key. Find out what makes you happy, and *try to do it*. Find out what is bothering you, and *try to resolve it*, and let it go once and for all. Your life will be so much more enjoyable as a result, and the excess weight will be much easier to lose.

If You Don't Already Have One, Get a Life!

Sometimes when I hear about the latest computer worm/virus launched, I often think, "People should just get a life!" Why are people so bored, with such a lack of positive focus that they would spend days/weeks/months working on something that will cause others harm? They get no money or positive attention for doing this, and they could go to jail for it! *What's the point?* Obviously these people have talent, the ability to focus and a lot of dedication/determination— *why not put it to good use?* I guess that's what I mean by get a life—using the talents, abilities and time that you have to do something positive for yourself or others. "Getting a life" means you are using your talents to make the world a better place. "Getting a life" also means you have positive things to focus on, which means you will rarely be bored…

People, especially children, need to be a part of something bigger than themselves in order to be productive and constructive. This is why children involved in organized sports, bands, clubs, or organizations *usually* get into less trouble than those left to their own devices—they have a focus other than just themselves. Being a part of something or working toward a goal raises your self-esteem and gives you less time to sit around watching TV, eating, and/or feeling sorry for yourself. You wake up every morning with a goal or something you look forward to doing. That is one of the keys to feeling fulfilled—having something worthwhile to do, making your mark or contribution to the world around you. *You feel better about yourself.*

At the height of my overweight teenage years, I would constantly tell my mother I was bored. Sure I would read, watch television, and listen to music, but my boredom stemmed from not having a passion/interest to focus on. The old adage is true—an idle mind is the devil's workshop because when we don't have something positive to focus on we wind up doing things we may not want to do such as drugs, excessive drinking, and, yes, you guessed it—*overeating*. When I was bored I used to watch TV and eat most of the night. Was I hungry? *No*. Does the body care why we are eating? *No*. So the laws of physiology dictate that the calories are treated the same way—*the extra ones turn into fat*. At that time, my only focus was how unhappy and lonely I was. I didn't really have a life at that point, but in my efforts to get one, I realized that I have a valuable place in this world. I actually have work to do. *So do you...* If you find you have a lot of time to feel sorry for yourself or you tend to be bored a lot, it could mean you need to find a constructive activity to put *your* hands to—some good work that *you* can do.

Can you relate to any of this? Everyone's life is different, so for some people this section may not be relevant but, if you are one of the few people who can relate, let's commit to working on getting you a life or the life that you want. No one can tell you what that life should be, and it does not have to be some noble humanitarian effort. We don't have to save the world, but there is something for each of us to do to help make it a better place. Some people might think my earlier projects on hair care were trivial, but the e-mails I received thanking me for the help let me know differently. No one can tell you what your life's focus should be—**the only rule is that it should be positive and help others.** Even if you enjoy working in your yard (e.g., mowing, weeding, planting, etc...), you are making your neighborhood look better, and I am sure your neighbors appreciate it! So don't worry about anyone else, just do what you do, and work to create the life you want.

Putting Your Best Foot Forward

Did you know that the world treats you the way you act/carry yourself? All people were created equally in terms of worth/value, but we are not all treated equally. Although it is wrong, people often treat us the way we act or appear. If we appear timid, lacking in self-confidence, looking down instead of making eye contact, people may make assumptions that could cause them to miss or not realize our full talent, intelligence, or worth. So, when we change the way we carry ourselves, it often changes the way people treat us for the better. However, the other, more important, benefit has to do with the way we view ourselves. The more confident we act, *the more confident we feel*, and the more we will want to do and accomplish (e.g., apply for a new job, start a new business, end an abusive relationship, make new friends, etc.). I do realize this is often easier said than done... However, to live life to its fullest, it must be done... To make the process easier I have come up with a few things you can do to get started on your personal path to having more self-confidence and greater self-esteem:

1. Stand up straight, suck in your stomach (or gut, as they used to say in the military), hold your head high, and walk as if you have already accomplished your grandest dreams.

2. Look everyone you meet in the eye and smile, or say hello to almost anyone who makes eye contact with you. *I think making eye contact with people is one of the most powerful things you can do.* It is an act of confidence—even if you don't feel it, this is one time where you should fake it until you make it. When I was younger, I didn't always feel like making eye contact with people, especially those who dressed better, had more money, looked better or who I thought might have looked down on me. Because I did not want to see those thoughts expressed in someone's eyes, and I was not proud of who I was, I looked down instead. This simple act said to anyone who may have thought they were better/better off, "*I agree with you. You are right. You are better.*"

Guess what? That's how many people treated me then—*as if they were better.* However, as I matured and started to see myself as God sees me, as one of His children, with immense possibilities and great worth, I decided to stop looking down... I don't care if you are a king or a person on the street, if you look my way, I will make eye contact with you, and nine times out of time, I will smile and say hello—it has become a habit. I think this says to the world, I am worthy of your acknowledgement whether you want to give it or not, and "you" are worthy of mine. This one change helped *change* my posture, my thoughts, my attitude and the way others interact with me forevermore. It also helped improve my confidence and ultimately my circumstances (e.g., career, financial, relationships, *and* weight).

3. Speak up. Make sure everyone can hear you when you are sharing an idea or trying to make a point. Never say "*never mind*" or "*oh, nothing*." **Your ideas have value, and so do you.** Even if your idea is not the best idea presented, people who may have never noticed you before may begin to *really see you* for the first time. This helps get us noticed, as we all should be. We are not invisible, *no one is*. However, we can sometimes be tricked into *acting* invisible (e.g., looking down, speaking in a low, weak voice, etc.) which is a terrible waste. So make a decision today that you will never fade into the woodwork because of your size or any other characteristic you are not proud of. When given a chance to be heard, take it, and let the world hear what they have been missing. **You deserve respect. You deserve to be acknowledged. You have gifts and talents to offer this world.**

4. If you are in a relationship where a person is calling you fat or other hurtful, disrespectful names—*get out*. If you are in friendships where you are being mistreated—*get out*. If you are in a job situation where you are not respected, abused, or devalued, and you don't see it changing—plan an exit strategy, and move on as soon as possible! Being in toxic environments can contribute to low self-esteem or emotional distress, which can cause us to reach for food. Don't let anyone break your spirit. Don't let anyone make you feel bad about yourself—I don't care if it is your mother, father, sister, brother, etc. *No one should be allowed to do this to you.* Stand up for yourself, even if it means temporarily distancing yourself from the person/people. You don't have to blow up and completely sever the relationship, but you could say, "*I don't appreciate how you are talking to me. It needs to change.*" Give them a chance to fix it before distancing yourself, and based on the results you see, do what you need to do. *Your esteem and mental well-being are too important.*

5. Accentuate your positive features, through makeup, clothes, accessories, or shoes. Wear clothes that make you feel good about yourself. One

way I trick myself into feeling confident during important meetings or presentations is by dressing up in my favorite suit and heels (*even if the meeting is business casual*). I also show up early so I feel prepared. This helps me appear confident even if I don't feel it 100 percent, and it can help you too.

6. Be bold even if you don't always feel it. Take risks, and step up for tasks that you might not ordinarily. Stretch yourself. Strive for excellence, and when you succeed, you will see what I already know—*you are capable of doing a lot more than what you might even believe.* However, you will never know unless you put yourself out there, but once you do, your confidence will soar higher and higher.

7. Make every effort to "*do unto others as you would have them do unto you.*" Treat people the way you want to be treated (e.g., be nice and polite, go heavy on honest compliments—if someone looks nice, tell them, if they did a good job, let them know, etc.). Remember, what you put out, usually comes back to you.

8. Adopt a theme song (e.g., Patti Labelle's *New Attitude* or *New Day*, Mariah Carey's *Make it Happen,* or Mary J Blige's *Just Fine*, etc...) and listen to it frequently. *Make it Happen* was my theme song during my last year of college, and it worked wonders for my morale. I listened to it every time I headed out to the computer science classes that were kicking my butt or to the Financial Aid Office to ask for help. Guess what? It helped keep me going.

I know what you are thinking... These tips sound almost too simple to have any chance of ever helping you change your situation, right? Well, I am here to tell you, they can help get you in the right frame of mind to *GO OUT* and *DO*—to go out and get that new job you want, to stand up to people at work who may be underestimating you or holding you back, or talk to the cute guy you keep running into. Implementing these tips can help give you that extra oomph to take you to the next level in almost any area of your life and get you feeling good about yourself. And guess what? One of the keys to getting your weight under control is you feeling good about Y-O-U. Trust me, **you must feel good about yourself BEFORE you lose the weight**; otherwise, you may get to a healthy weight, but you may not be any happier.

In fact, I heard women on Oprah talking about problems they experienced after losing weight (e.g., *alcohol, drug addictions, promiscuity, etc.*). I think this is the part they neglected—they were at a healthy weight, but they still didn't feel good about themselves. I don't know about you, but going through the trouble of losing weight, and then not being able to enjoy the accomplishment is no fun to me. This is why I put this chapter before the ones on exercise and eating. I don't know about you, but I want it all—a healthy body, mind, and spirit. *I hope that is your goal as well.* Once it is, the whole weight loss process will be much easier, and the results will be more long-lasting.

Managing Your Stress Levels

Here is the final piece to my *get-your-mind-right* strategy. Have you noticed when you are stressed, uptight or under major pressure, you want to reach for something—a *Coke*, chips, cookies, a candy bar, ice cream, cake, anything bad (e.g., never fruit or vegetables)? For the average person overwhelming stress levels may only happen a few times a month or week, which may not wreck your normal eating routine. However, what if you allow your stress levels to build where you feel overwhelmed on a daily basis or consistently throughout the day? This will have you reaching for snacks left and right—accepting treats offered at work, visiting vending machines, keeping a private stash of goodies, etc. As a result, your efforts to have healthier eating habits will fail, and all of the appetite suppressants in the world won't be able to help you. You can indulge in this foolishness occasionally, but doing it consistently will undermine any weight loss/maintenance efforts. So, the root cause, stress or feelings of being overwhelmed, must be managed. Here are a few ideas to help you do just that:

1. Listen to any type of music that soothes you (e.g., classical, jazz, etc.). Sometimes when I feel under stress I turn on classical, old-school rap or disco music (*I know this is a strange mix*), and I listen or dance based on my mood. I feel better almost immediately. This is therapeutic for the body, mind and spirit. It allows us to momentarily check out from the cares of everyday life, and sometimes that is all that's needed—*just a moment*. In the era of iPods, docking stations, and portable speakers, we can listen to the

music we love, wherever and whenever we want. So hopefully this is an easy change to implement.

2. Relax doing any activity that you enjoy: reading magazines or motivational books (e.g., the Bible, authors like Jack Canfield and Mark Victor Hansen, etc.), knitting or sewing, playing an instrument, painting, etc. *Just do something that YOU want to do.*

3. Play a sport or exercise—it can be something as simple as a walk around the block.

4. You could even take a few moments to yourself when you get home from work to just lie back on the bed or a chair with your eyes closed to decompress.

5. Some of us need more help to relax and let go of the stresses of the day, so deep breathing exercises (slowly inhale through your nose, hold and exhale slowly through your mouth), meditation, or prayer might be even more helpful.

6. Take a moment to vent to a friend or loved one. It can be over lunch, coffee or dinner. However, it works even better if you walk and talk. Even if the person can't walk with you, you can talk to them on the phone while *you* walk. In fact, I've walked while ranting/venting. Believe me, I felt a lot better when I got home.

7. Cuddling with your special someone (laying in the bed for thirty minutes while talking and hugging on a Saturday or Sunday morning with my husband can eradicate a whole week's worth of stress for both of us from work, maintaining our household, managing kids, etc.). Doing this gives our whole weekend a more positive, less stressful feel. Nothing may actually change, but our perception/attitude is a whole lot better. You could also cuddle with one of your children for as long as they will allow, and let them tell you goofy jokes or talk about something crazy that happened at school.

No children or special someone? What about playing with or stroking your pet's fur? No pets? Oh well, not to worry, you could do what I do when I am really upset… Lie in bed (sometimes after a good cry), and talk to God. I am so glad He doesn't smite people because

I would certainly be smitten, as I have often fussed, complained, and asked Him why this/why not that. I also thank Him and ask for help. Basically I talk to Him like a small child might talk to a parent. I usually lie on my side as if my head is in His lap, and He is actually stroking my hair like a parent might. *Crazy, huh?* You might think so, but many times I can feel His presence, and I am comforted, especially when I've done this while waiting in exam rooms to hear the results of a follow-up mammogram, sonogram, or an echocardiogram. I don't know if it is a coincidence, but I have always gotten good results when I have done this, and I always walk away feeling better and closer to God. See what works for you, *and do it!*

These seven steps can certainly help you better manage the everyday stresses in your life, helping you to avoid some of the pitfalls of stress-related overeating. However, there are other steps that could be taken as well to help you avoid or minimize unnecessary stress so you don't feel overwhelmed as often. Sometimes we can become punch-drunk from everything that comes our way during the course of a day. As the old saying goes, "*When it rains it pours.*" While this may be the case at times, would you agree that all stressful situations do not have to be handled all at once? All fires do not have to be put out at the same time, right? With this in mind, I think we would be better off if we pick our stress battles more carefully, and save some of them for another day. How do we do this? Well, here are a few of the ideas I have started practicing:

1. Do not open mail at night, especially on weekend nights. I only open mail on weekday mornings—*when I can do something about it if there is a problem.* I used to open mail when I got home in the evenings, but what happens when there is a billing error or a payment that was lost in the mail? What if I receive a letter from a collection agency regarding an account that was fraudulently opened in my name (*I have been the victim of identity theft multiple times*) or a bad account opened by someone with the same name? Because I *used* to be listed in the phone book, I would be the person agencies tracked down for accounts opened by other people with the same name. Of course I would open these letters at night...

Do you know how many times I wished I never opened those mails? I usually stewed all night about how I would resolve various problems the next day (e.g., calling people to prove that I was not the person they were looking for, preparing yet another fraud packet, etc.). Were these all matters that needed to be addressed? Of course, but what could I do about them at night other than drive myself crazy? Was there anyone I could call then to discuss/resolve it? No, of course not, but I let it add unnecessary stress to an already action-packed evening with kids who needed to be fed, homework that needed to be checked, things that needed to be washed/cleaned, etc. Issues that may come in the mail can stress us out for hours at night, but they can usually be resolved in less than fifteen minutes in the morning. So put the mail aside until then. Then, with the time saved, take a nice relaxing bath, and take your butt to bed!

2. Do not open e-mails or check voice mails that have to do with work in the evening. I usually save voice mails for the morning if I haven't checked them by 4:00 in the afternoon. It is basically the same story... If I can't do anything about it, why add that stress to the evening? I have even instructed my husband not to ask me any questions about business or mention anything business-related that will trouble me after dinner. Only tell me about situations/problems when I can actually do something about them. Otherwise, it is a complete waste of my mental and emotional energy, as well as the little downtime I may get in an evening. Some things really can keep until the morning. However, the chain e-mails that warn/scare us (e.g., ones on the dangers of bottled water, plastic bottles, etc.) may need to be avoided indefinitely. You will be surprised at how much *minimizing brain clutter* can help. Try it and see!

3. Make the most of Caller ID by screening all home phone calls in the evening (*my cell phone is usually turned off*). Because I am focused on the kids and *essential* tasks (e.g., cooking, exercise, etc.), I selectively answer our phone. I usually don't answer it as I am preparing/eating dinner. I tend to let calls go into voice mail, and I return them the next day. This is probably why my husband and I don't have a lot of friends! We value

our downtime in the evenings, and we try to protect it as it makes sense. You should protect yours as much as possible too.

4. Do not schedule routine physicals, mammograms or other serious screening tests right before a vacation if you can help it. Once I scheduled a mammogram a week before my family's summer vacation, and *of course* the reading came back abnormal, and I had to schedule a follow-up mammogram. So I had another mammogram right before leaving, and *of course*, I had to wait for the results while I was on my trip. If I had waited to have the procedure *AFTER* my vacation, the results would have been the same—a biopsy (Praise the Lord, it was nothing serious). However, the cloud that hung over my head during that vacation would not have been there, and my family would have had my undivided attention. So now my annual mammograms are scheduled *AFTER* our family vacation and *AFTER* my wedding anniversary! Also, my annual physical is now in early January, *AFTER* Christmas and New Year's Day.

I cannot tell you when to schedule your appointments because I know we can't always control these things, but when given a choice, maybe you could try to schedule them based on what is going on in your life. Does your physical/exam/test have to be scheduled the day before your birthday, vacation, or your big presentation at work? I say not if you can help it! Sometimes we do have choices about these things. So I make every effort to keep the cares of this life in manageable chunks by selectively scheduling my appointments. While I wait, my family has become accustomed to hearing me say, *"It'll be all right."* Meaning that whatever it is will keep until I can get to it, and I am not going to let it stress me out in the meantime. As a result, we get to enjoy the good times of life (e.g., birthdays, vacations, evenings at home joking around, etc.) with a free mind. I think this goes a long way toward keeping us from becoming overwhelmed, and it creates a happier home life. Maybe it can work for you too... *I think it can, but use sound judgment/discretion when putting things off.*

5. **Learn to say no.** This is especially important if you have kids or a stressful job. Because we are all so busy these days, having downtime to regroup and recover is essential to our mental and emotional

well-being. *So being able to say no to requests / demands placed on our time, as needed, may be the only way to get the downtime we need to preserve our sanity.* It seems like many of us are afraid to say no to requests for our time (e.g., meetings to discuss items already discussed, invites to events/places you don't feel like going to, baking cookies you are too tired to bake, taking your kids to extra practices/ scrimmages/unnecessary trips to the mall, last-minute plans just sprung on you, etc.). No more! *You must decide what is most important to you. Then, do as many of those things as you can. However, there must be time left for meals, exercise, relaxation, quality time with loved ones, and a good night's sleep. Any task left over? Delegate it, or just say no!*

You can't do it all, and let's be honest, *you don't want to. So stop trying!* At some point you have to say, **"This is not what I want to do with my time right now."** Stop. *No explanation or guilt required.* Some days you will volunteer or say "yes," but **not every time.** Other people feel free to tell us "no," and we accept it and move on. *The world won't end when we say "no."* I know some people may be annoyed, mad or disappointed, *but they will live*, and **they will get over it, and move on!**

We all need priorities and boundaries that should be observed as we decide how to spend our time. *Kids too.* As an example, I asked my oldest son if he *really* wanted to do what was required to play football (e.g., entire month of August practicing five nights a week, from 6:00-8:00 p.m., and three nights a week from 6:00–8:00 p.m. in September and October, *which includes Friday nights*). He said, "No." I was so glad because I didn't want to make the time commitment, but I would have for him... Some families love it, and I say more power to them, but for now, *we said no.* Friday is a day to decompress, where we get to do what we enjoy (e.g., kids play in the basement, I enjoy a *Red Bull* and watch a movie, my husband hangs out with friends, etc.). Some people think we are crazy when I tell them we chose this over football, but I think *we all must choose what is most important to us* as individuals/families (*I choose quality of life*), and *other things are cut loose.* Remember it is better to do a few things well and be happy, *instead of doing many things in a less than excellent way and being unhappy or stressed out.*

6. Try to find ways to save time and reduce your efforts so you have more free time. It is very hard to decompress if you don't have a free moment to think or breathe. I mean there are so many tasks for us to do and be involved in that we are often running all over creation (e.g., looking for gifts, clothes, things for the house, etc.). I don't know about you, but the time spent on these little to-do items adds up and can drive you crazy as they are added to your existing list of tasks. As an example, one organization I recently joined required me to wear white shoes to a ceremony. Do you know how hard it is for someone who wears a ten to find a cute pair of white shoes? It would probably require me to go to multiple stores, waste hours of effort, time, and gas. This one task could have taken weeks! Who has that kind of time? I know I don't!

This one task helped me to decide I would no longer waste time running all over creation looking for hard-to-find items. What did I do? I went to the Internet and Googled the words "white pumps" and "Guess," and *guess* what happened? I found the most wonderful patent leather pumps, with a metallic gold heel, under $100, and with free shipping! What could have taken weeks was handled in an hour. As a result, I now look online for wedding gifts, items for the house, clothes, etc. This philosophy opened up a whole new world for me—I am now more productive, my overall stress is minimized, and I am less likely to overload on junk-food...

7. Accept the fact that there are only so many things you can accomplish in one day, and GO TO SLEEP! *You cannot do everything.* Something may have to give. Being well rested helps us to be healthier, in a better mood, more productive during actual work hours, and less tempted to eat junk at night. This is the hardest piece of advice for me to follow, but my body tends to shut down when I am overly tired. Sometimes you just need to go to bed. **Do what you can, and save the rest for another day.**

Can you believe that many of the triggers that cause us to overeat are linked to how we handle the cares of our lives (many of the items mentioned above)? Removing some of the extra stuff helps to free our minds so we can focus on what's really important, allowing us to do more of the things in life that bring us joy. I think you will be amazed at how your eating habits change when you focus on what is really important to you and put your health and quality of life at the top of the list. Believe it or not, this is a key step to losing weight and keeping it off… Remember, the less uptight and overwhelmed you are, the less likely you are to overeat.

~

Chapter 6

Request & Receive Help (Step 4)

There is a big difference between wanting a change and wanting to *make* a change in your life. Many people want to lose weight, like I did, but they don't actually want to change anything. Are you prepared to eat cereal, oatmeal, or something equally as healthy for breakfast a few days a week? *Most would say no.* Are you prepared to include walking in your lifestyle a few times a week? Again, many would say no. Now if you asked those same people would they like to lose weight or feel healthier? You would hear a resounding "Yes." So why is it that we want change, but we don't want *to* change? Well, speaking from experience, I can say the answer is easy. People are naturally lazy and often resistant to change, *myself included.*

Even so, that doesn't mean we can't change. As I mentioned before, insanity has been defined as doing the same thing over and over again, expecting a different result. So if you want to change your weight, or any other area of your life for that matter, you must be willing to make changes, *to do something different.* However, making the necessary changes, or doing something different, could be out of your area of expertise or beyond what you are capable of doing on your own. This is why books are written, and support groups are formed. Because we can't always reach our goals on our own, especially where losing weight and getting fit are concerned. These are often areas where we may need to request or ask for help.

Exhaust All Possibilities

I know the whole ask for help thing is hard for some of us. *I know it is for me*, but from time to time, we do need a little help from our friends and loved ones to help us reach our health, fitness, and weight loss goals. As an example, a husband may need his wife's help in preparing healthier meals; kids may need this same help from their parents; parents may need this type of help from a nutritionist, other parents, family members or a class; moms may need help with tasks around the house to free up time for exercise; or wives/husbands may need their spouse's help getting started on a consistent exercise program (walks are a lot nicer with two people). I was amazed at how quickly the extra pounds started to come off for me and my family when we exercised and ate healthier together. I believe it is important for families to adopt the philosophy that when one person has a weight problem (e.g., husband, wife, child, etc.), *the WHOLE family has a problem*, and *it must be dealt with as a family*. If one person needs to run, we ***all*** need to run or walk along with them if necessary. When one person needs exercise, *we all exercise*. In fact, when I want to drop a few pounds, my sons are (*sometimes*) happy to play basketball, tennis, kickball, or any physical activity I want at the time, even walking to parks, stores, restaurants or to the post office. Good health and physical fitness should be a family affair, and if our families don't offer, *we must ask*.

Including my family in my exercise activities serves three purposes: 1) It makes exercise/physical activity fun for me and not a chore; 2) It allows us to spend quality time together, where we get to laugh and talk; and 3) It is a major stress reliever for all of us. However, for those of you who do not have a family unit to rely on for help in this area or who do not have a family that is willing/able to help, do not fear. You could ask friends, neighbors, a church group, or colleagues for help wherever you may need it (e.g., to get weekly tennis/racquetball games started, attend aerobic or dance classes, swim, walk or do anything physical that does not involve excessive eating). If none of these are options for you, and you struggle taking on the commitment of losing weight/exercising on your own, you may be a good candidate for a support group (formal or informal). I think this is why weight loss clinics have become so popular across the country—because many of us are looking for help.

While I understand the appeal and the popularity of clinics/groups, **I do not believe this is something the average person should pay for**, especially when your biggest support team/help could be in your house, neighborhood, church, school, or office. *You just may not have found them yet.* You never know, your support/help could come from unlikely sources. In fact, I used to rollerblade with our neighbor's pre-teen son! He didn't have anyone to skate with, and I had just learned. So, with his parents' blessing, we would skate together in our neighborhood. You may have to get creative, but the more likely you are to involve your family, friends, or a group in your activities, the more likely you are to enjoy physical activity **and** get the encouragment you need during weak moments. As a result, you will be more likely to continue with your undertaking for a lifetime, not just for a week or a month. Even if you don't have someone who can/is willing to exercise with you, you may know someone who will listen as you talk out your fears, thoughts and challenges, as well as encourage you and praise you as you get closer to your goal. Don't underestimate the power of a support group/team of people who are rooting for you. However, what happens if you don't have that *even after* you have asked for help? Well, I have an answer for that too…

When All Else Fails

When I was trying to lose weight as a young adult (from about thirteen to nineteen), I seriously can't recall anyone that was available to help me in terms of getting into shape or listening to any of the things that concerned me. I remember asking my mom to teach me to play basketball (she played in high school) or to play with me, but after she said no so many times, I finally stopped asking. I also begged her for a bike for years so I had an activity I could do by myself and that would get me out of the house, but she was scared that I would get run over by a car. *This could have been related to the fact that a friend I had when I was five was killed by a car when she ran out into the street.* Maybe on some level I understood, but for the most part, I was very frustrated, especially since it was just the two of us, so there were not too many other people to ask for help. Also, as I mentioned before, I grew up feeling that no one really cared about me or the things that concerned me, and I just never felt that there was someone rooting for me. As a result, I really felt as if *I had exhausted all possibilities, and all else had failed.*

I know I did not consciously think or say this, but at some point you have a choice of giving up or trying something radically different. I think these were the times during my childhood/teen years where God seemed to be the only one I had not gone to for help and had not been disappointed by. So why not give Him a try as my life/weight loss support buddy? I felt like I had no one else. Also, as I mentioned earlier in the book, I had more than a few struggles I was trying to work through, so I really needed help. People had always told me that *He* could do anything, so my little problems should have been nothing for Him to handle, right? What did I have to lose *other than weight?*

I am sure this may seem crazy to some of you, and many of you may laugh, especially atheists and agnostics, but when you have no one else, I have found God to be a safe place to fall/lean when life gets hard. As a young woman, I must admit that I didn't know if He was real. I only had the word of people who told me about Him. So my attitude started off as, *"Why not?"* After all, what other options did I have as pressure mounted, my weight started increasing, and there was no one who was able or willing to help? *None.* So I exercised *the God-option* as a last resort, and guess what? I finally got the help I needed (*see Wake-up Call #1*), and I am sure you can too. *Fortunately He doesn't seem to mind being a last resort option!* So I am not telling you *who* to ask, but I am letting you know that this option has worked for me time and time again. Take this time to think of who you might request help from, and be ready to receive it!

꩜

Chapter 7

Rev Up Your Engine & Revolutionize Your Activity (Step 5)

Now that we have gone through the emotional and mental baggage that usually contributes to excess weight, we can move on to the tangible things that you can do to get the ball rolling in a physical sense. I know I put you through a lot of hoops to get here, but think about it, how many exercise programs have you started with the best of intentions only to grow tired of them and give up after just a few weeks? If it were really so straightforward and easy, you would have lost the weight and kept it off years ago, right? So there is a method to my madness, and because we addressed the emotional and the mental first, I think you have a better chance of finding an exercise and eating regimen that you can stick with for the long haul.

Because I am a person who can get overwhelmed and shut down when I have to make too many changes at once, my approach to weight loss and life in general has become one where I take things one step at a time or one day at a time, whichever the case may be. This is why I decided to *focus on the exercise portion first and tackle the whole food / eating thing later.* It may surprise you to find out that this one-step-at-a-time philosophy can help keep you from becoming overwhelmed and giving up. In case I haven't said it before, **giving up is not** *an option.* Also, as I mentioned before, *you didn't gain the weight overnight, so you cannot expect to lose it overnight either.*

With that said, let's toss aside all of the extremes that you used to associate with exercising to lose weight. Can we agree that the only thing being extreme does is frustrate us? Things done to the extreme cannot be continued successfully for the long haul, and that's what we want—***long-term success***. So let's start off by throwing all of the "*have to's*" out of the window. *We don't have to jog/run. We don't have to wake up every morning at 5:00 a.m. to exercise for an hour. We don't have to go to a gym every night after work.* We don't *have to* do these things to get to or maintain a healthy weight, and boy am I glad! Can you believe that there are millions of people around the world at healthy weights that never formally "exercise"? It's true, and even more surprisingly, millions of Americans in years past never officially *exercised*, yet their rates of obesity, heart disease, and high blood pressure were significantly lower than ours. How is this possible when we are living in one of the most modern and technologically advanced societies ever in existence? We must be doing something wrong...

Getting To the Heart of the Matter

What are we doing wrong? Well, for one, I think many of us have settled into our sedentary lifestyles (e.g., working long hours, driving everywhere, *sitting and watching* our kids play sports, watching more and more TV while eating and drinking more and more as we sit on the couch, etc.), and *we have gotten very comfortable*. Don't get me wrong, this is not a judgment, just a statement of fact. Any fingers I point at you are also pointed at me, believe me. When you look at how driven we are from our jobs to professional/religious/social affiliations, from kids' activities to even caring for our yards and homes, our predicament is definitely understandable. I believe many of us are excessively busy, overwhelmed and tired, and we feel our lives are out of balance, and in many cases they are...

Could that be why we drive everywhere; why we don't even want to get up to change a channel; why we call, e-mail or text-message people even if they are within walking distance in another cube; why we prefer elevators and escalators to stairs (even if they are right next to the escalator); why we don't play games like kickball, baseball, or touch football with our kids and instead give them video games to play while we watch TV? Our lives have become a hard juggling act, and I can clearly see why we tend to throw our hands up and say, *"Forget it!"* when it comes to trying to do it all **and** still include exercise and healthy eating. To come to our defense, I think we, *with the help of diet book authors and weight loss professionals*, have made losing weight and eating healthier way too hard. If you look at most of the plans for losing weight and eating healthier, they seem to be all-or-nothing propositions, and because the *"all"* seems to be too much, most of us have resigned ourselves to just do nothing. I think this is one of the reasons our weight has started to spiral out of control. *We are starting to give up...*

Even though the situation is literally reaching a critical mass, all is really not lost. As you continue reading you will find that losing weight and keeping it off forever is not as hard as you once thought it to be. I never thought I would ever be saying this, but it is actually pretty simple once you get started on a one-step-at-a-time, one-day-at-a-time plan that is based on your lifestyle as well as *your* likes and dislikes. The goal of the next chapter is to help you do just that. As your plan evolves, be sure to keep it as **simple** as you can, make it *fun* whenever possible, and be **consistent**. *This is the secret to your long-term success—a plan that is simple, fun, and consistent.* However, before you can come up with your simple and fun plan, you will need to acknowledge a few basic principles...

Back to Basics

The basic principle of weight loss 101, as we all know, is *you must burn more calories than you take in over time*. In fact, just to lose a pound you need to burn an additional 3,500 calories over time, and even though I don't want you to sit around counting the calories you take in or burn, those are the facts. I will admit, it does sound like a lot of effort to burn just one pound, which is why I keep repeating that the weight wasn't gained overnight, so you can't expect to lose it overnight. However, there is no reason to lose hope. Because even if you did nothing more than burn 100 extra calories a day through exercise (e.g., a simple walk) or by using mustard instead of mayonnaise or drinking water instead of soda, do you know you could lose more than ten pounds in a year?

That is the real secret to weight loss—*burning more calories than you take in*. Only if it were as easy to implement as it is to say!

Well to some extent, maybe it is... To burn more calories than you take in, you literally gotta get up and move something every day—*your arms, your legs, your butt...* It doesn't matter *what* you are moving, but you gotta move *SOMETHING!* However, you don't have to be constrained by those pesky "*have-to's*" I mentioned earlier. What if I told you that you could make a radical difference in your body/weight just by taking a quick walk after dinner in the evenings? Just a measly fifteen- to thirty-minute walk is enough to make a major difference, especially if you walk with a sense of purpose and you do it at least four or five times a week. Each walk would count toward burning the 3,500 calories necessary to lose a pound. *The more you do, the more you lose.* It is just like saving money or investing—the same way pennies saved consistently can add up to big gains, the extra calories you burn on a daily basis can definitely add up to big losses in calories *and* weight.

Creating a Lifestyle of Movement

This puts a slightly different spin on the whole exercise thing, huh? Exercise does not have to be formal or extreme—*it just has to be consistent*. Fifty years ago people didn't flock to gyms in droves like we do today, yet they were in better shape than we are. Also people in many other countries do not have formal exercise programs, yet they are often healthier, weigh less, and live longer than we do. I think one of the reasons is because *moving* is a way of life for them. I have heard that the French, who frequently indulge in rich foods, tend not to have the same obesity rates that we do, and their rates of heart disease and hypertension are lower. It would seem that their more active lifestyles allow them to eat more and go to the gym less. They usually walk more and center social gatherings around physical activities, namely walking to restaurants and other outings. We *used* to do that, but we do it less and less to the point where people are even surprised to see neighbors walking to and from the store. In fact, there have been a number of times where people have offered me rides as I was walking home from the grocery store. I would jokingly yell, "*Thanks, but that would defeat the whole purpose!*"

This mind-set is understandable because we have become lazy, and unfortunately we are getting lazier by the minute. Gym memberships are popular in the United States, but our general level of activity has never been lower, and we have never been heavier than we are now. It is time to reverse this trend before it is too late, and one of the ways we can do this is by creating a *lifestyle of movement*. Don't get me wrong, I do believe that sticking to a formal exercise program is probably the best way for most people in our society to get and stay in shape. However, I also believe formal routines are hard to stick with over time unless you *really* enjoy a particular activity. I tell you if I didn't *truly* enjoy walking, I would struggle to do it on a daily basis. On the other hand, I don't enjoy swimming (*I am not good at the whole breathing thing or treading water*), biking, aerobics, or running, which is why you will rarely see me doing these things. These activities feel more like work than fun, especially running (*my knees tend to hurt*). Some may view it as fun, and I say more power to them, but it is not for me, at least not for the long-term. If it is for you, I say, "*Run on, my friend. Run on.*"

Now what if I want to see some of the same benefits as women who are running for miles while I am only walking about thirty to forty-five minutes a day? I obviously need to supplement my activity levels. Naturally, walking can't be all that I do, especially if I am trying to lose weight or majorly improve my fitness level. This is where the whole concept of creating a lifestyle of movement comes in—*the systematic, consistent effort to move and do more, even as technological advances are constantly making it easier and more logical for us to do less and less.* I think you will be amazed at how much this extra effort can supplement the results of our existing or *budding* exercise routines. So with all of this said, how do we create this whole lifestyle of movement? Although there is no set answer, it is definitely a question worth asking. It is easier than you may think, but it may not be so obvious where you would think of it yourself… For this reason, I have outlined a What-if model that can help get you started and literally rev up your engine:

What If …

1. You took the stairs at your office EVERY morning instead of the elevator and used the bathroom on a different floor in your building or house, taking the stairs each time?

2. You got up every half hour to walk around your office or home? Ask questions in person, drop off work or requested items, get water, just make up excuses to get up.

3. You walked to pick up your lunch instead of driving or you walked after eating lunch?

4. After dinner you put on your favorite dance music and danced like you did when you were younger a few nights a week? Make it easier by creating a playlist on your iPod specifically for this purpose.

5. You walked to Starbucks to pick up your weekend coffee/drink/treat?

6. You parked at the opposite end of the mall/plaza from the store where you plan to shop and walked from one end to the other in the course of your shopping?

7. You walked while you wait for your children to finish soccer/football/ cheerleading practice *instead of* talking to the other moms or reading in your car?

8. You bought a treadmill and walked, jogged, or ran on it during your favorite TV show(s) in the evening (e.g., *The Celebrity Apprentice*, *America's Next Top Model*, *American Idol* or *Lost*—these are some of the shows I have watched while walking)? The time, speed, or intensity of the workout doesn't matter. Just work at your own pace while you enjoy a show.

9. You took a short walk every night after dinner? Around the neighborhood, the block or even your house—*just get out and go!*

10. You walked your kids to a friend's house to play instead of driving them?

11. You are at home in the morning and you walked your small children to school a few times a week? This would help you *and them* be more active, *and* you get to talk.

12. You took your kids to a skating rink and taught them to skate or they taught you, and then you all spent some time skating? Skating could become a family activity.

13. The whole family walked to the grocery store, shopped, and carried the bags home?

14. You decided to stop driving to places that are walking distance from your house (e.g., post office, stores, restaurants, pool, etc.)? Want a sub from
· Subway or forgot something at the grocery store? *Walk to get it!* Don't burn gas, burn calories instead!

15. You took a class for hiking, rollerblading, tennis, swimming, Latin dancing, and you liked it enough to include the newly learned activity in your weekly schedule?

16. You scheduled a standing kickball game with your kids every week? It could also be tennis, basketball, or softball.

17. You bought a bike and started riding it with your kids, spouse, a friend, or by yourself?

18. You told the kids they can have Chinese food, but you *all* have to walk to the restaurant (as long as it is within one to two miles, and it is safe of course), or they have to play outside while you walk to pick it up?

19. You made it your goal to run up and down the stairs in your house as often as you can? Try taking items from the basement to the top level a few times a day.

20. You did calisthenics whenever you have an opportunity (e.g., while you wait for the microwave to finish warming up an item)? Maybe start off with ten jumping jacks and push-ups in the morning, and then again at night.

21. You formed a walking group with people from your neighborhood, church, or work?

22. You volunteered to help out at a hospital/organization where there is a lot of walking?

23. You started participating in walks for causes (e.g., for the homeless, diabetes, breast cancer, cystic fibrosis, etc.)? Some are as short as a mile, and they have no time limit.

24. You turned on some of your favorite dance music and just started cleaning your house (e.g., vacuuming, sweeping, cleaning windows or walls, etc.)?

25. You and your spouse or a friend went to a mall, and you walked around as many of the levels as you can for an hour? Take the stairs as much as possible. You can window-shop, but it only counts as exercise if you walk with a sense of purpose.

26. You played a game with your spouse or kids (e.g., tennis, basketball, racquetball, Frisbee, tag, etc.) after dinner or on the weekend?

27. You pulled out one of the many exercise DVDs/tapes that may be collecting dust on a shelf and did a workout? Try a different one each week to see if you can find one that you want to do on a regular basis. I just recently started doing the *Perfect Shape Fat Blasting Routines* by Body Wisdom Media Inc.

(I have had it forever). The Boot Camp routines are fun even though I only do them occasionally.

28. You did a few high kicks like the *Rockettes* while you are watching TV, or you crouch down, touch the floor and jump as high as you can? *Then, do it again if you can.*

29. You did leg lifts or squats while you fill your glass with ice/water, wash dishes, or brush your teeth?

30. You played games like *Dance Pad Revolution* or *Wii Fit* (it even has yoga as well as cardio) with your kids, or by yourself, at least once a week?

I could go on and on, but I am sure you get the idea, and I bet you have ideas of your own by now. Bottom line: *find ways to make moving and being active fun and purposeful instead of just "exercise" or work.* I know my suggestions may seem too simple to make a difference, but they are viable ways to increase our daily activity levels and significantly reduce sedentary time (*time spent on the couch or behind a desk*). They also provide a perfect starting point if you have not been very active for a while, allowing you to gradually increase your activity level by engaging in less strenuous activities on a regular basis. In time, you may be able to engage in more strenuous activities, but for now the goal is just to get you moving more in general. This will automatically boost the number of calories you burn every day, and guess what? *Over time*, if you are consistently moving *and* engaging in at least one regular form of exercise, this will add up to BIG results on the scale, in the mirror, and in the way you feel!

Get Creative

Creating a lifestyle of movement is a good thing, and it should be a lifetime commitment whether you have a weight problem or not. Remember, we are not just exercising to lose weight... *We are exercising because the organs and systems in our bodies need it, and because it will help us live a longer, more enjoyable life.* Other benefits include: you will look younger, you won't suffer from as many ailments, you will be able to manage stress better, and when done consistently, you will ultimately lose, and/or maintain a healthy weight. For all of these reasons, **exercise is required.** *Whether you are trying to lose weight or not.* It is not optional. That's why I put this chapter before the ones on eating. However, the activity you choose is optional. *It does not have to be in a gym, and* *it does not have to be running.* Thank God! It could be dancing in your kitchen. In fact, I saw Kirstie Alley on *Oprah* talking about dancing her way to a seventy-five-pound weight loss. It was very confirming for me because I have been dancing in my kitchen and family room for years, for fun and exercise. Dancing may be a possibility for you as well. However, you won't know until you try. In the meantime, just pick an activity, and try to do it on a regular basis. *Your life, health, and waistline depend on it.*

After I had my first son, I did something daring: I took a rollerblading class. For Mother's Day I asked for a pair of skates and all of the essential safety gear, and I took a class through the county where I live. After the class, we started going to parks and parking areas where my husband would push our son in the stroller, and I would skate. Between the treadmill, rollerblades, and walking, I was able to work off the last twenty plus pounds of baby-weight. Thinking back, I remember tolerating the treadmill, but I *enjoyed* rollerblading. As I said before, this led me to skate with a kid from the neighborhood. We would skate up and down a street near our house. It was wonderful! I am sure his parents were happy because he was supervised and wasn't bored, but I was happy because I had found a fun way to get exercise and take a break from the stress of being a new mom. After a while the kid started knocking on our door to ask if *I could come out and play!*

Although this was funny, my eyes were forever open to the many ways we can fit a healthier lifestyle in and enjoy life to the fullest. It also enabled me to be a better mother to my children because it helped me to see that kids like it when adults play with them. In fact, some of the best exercise I have ever gotten is from running behind my children on their bikes or scooters, racing them, or playing kickball/basketball. They love it! It is also a way to connect, and it keeps them and *me* healthy. Playing tennis with them has also been good exercise for me. For the longest we didn't even worry about the score or rules. Our goal was just to have fun and get some exercise. Now that we keep score, and they have had lessons, I am lucky if I ever win a game. However, it doesn't matter if you win or lose—just running and hitting the ball back and forth can provide a good workout. So a big part of my regimen has been to try to find activities that I can do with the kids every week (getting harder as they get older and play sports), and the rest of the week I walk/jog, jump rope, do floor exercises and take the stairs as much as I can.

All of that to say, exercise is not an all-or-nothing proposition. You just need to make a decision and commitment to move as much as possible. Your exercise can be done all at once or intermittently throughout the day. Why not start off with walking ten to fifteen minutes a day, whenever you get a chance, for three days a week? Then later you could build up to thirty minutes of more intense walking at least five days a week. With this regimen you can burn one hundred to two hundred plus calories more per day. We should set a long-term goal to do at least thirty minutes or more of moderate-intensity physical activity on most, *preferably all*, days of the week. This regimen can be adapted to include other forms of physical activity (i.e., resistance/strength training), but walking is particularly attractive because it is low impact, most people can do it, and you can kinda ease into it. In addition to this, try to increase the "everyday" activities such as taking the stairs instead of the elevator, walking to lunch, etc. Doing this over time will help improve your fitness level so you can engage in more strenuous activities such as competitive sports and marathons if that is your goal. However, for now, you just need to make being active a habit.

Other Ways to Get Moving

I hope some of the suggestions and experiences I have shared so far have inspired you to get up and get moving. However, I am sure you have noticed by now that this chapter does not give pictures to show you how to exercise. *This was completely intentional…* Has any book ever *really* helped you exercise more by showing you pictures on how to exercise? In most cases, I am sure the answer is no. Books and magazines with pictures of people exercising line the shelves of every major book store, and many of us have videotapes/DVDs that show us how to exercise collecting dust in our entertainment centers. Be that as it may, the average American is still not exercising, so I am not going to waste your time *or mine* with pictures. Instead, I have a few ideas for you to consider/try that have worked for me and my family:

- Utilize free resources to get ideas on incorporating exercise into your everyday life such as www.nih.gov, www.cdc.gov/physicalactivity, www.

acefitness.org, and www.shapeup.org. On these sites I found ideas such as aiming for ten thousand steps a day (two thousand steps = a mile). Steps are tracked by a pedometer (can be found at sporting goods/discount stores), which helps you see how active/*inactive* you really are. If you are physically able *and* have your doctor's approval, this could be a program to try. However, just be sure to test the pedometer out in different spots on various outfits because if it is not placed right, it will not record your steps properly. It only works for me if I put it on the waistband of my shorts or pants. So be sure to test its placement each time you use it. This is just one of the many ideas you can find on these Web sites.

- Knock on some neighbors'/friends' doors and ask if other people in need of exercise can come out and play. Find someone, *anyone*—it can even be one of your neighbor's kids, or their dog, to join you for a quick walk/jog in the morning or after dinner. It doesn't matter *who*, but you are more likely to go if someone will go with you. I know somebody is asking, "What if it is cold or raining?" Well, in those cases, you can ask someone to take a ride to the mall, and you can do laps around the mall (no treats can be bought though—*you are there to walk!*). To get the most out of the workout, be sure to make things more challenging by running up the stairs from one level to the next as many times as you can. If the mall is too far, go to the grocery store and do laps—no one will care, especially if you are buying groceries too. *Just don't go there hungry.* Also, even if you can't find anyone to go with you, go alone—I do most of my walking alone.

If you don't want to go to those places, grab a coat and go outside—you burn a few more calories when it is cold anyway. *You can fit it in if you really want to.* What if none of those options is feasible on a given day? Hop on a treadmill or stationery bike if you have one. Put it in front of a TV, and go for it! You don't have any exercise equipment at home? OK, well do you have stairs? If so, run up and down your stairs as many times as you can. Just do what you *can* do. Whenever you can, as you are able, make excuses to run—pretend like you are in a rush, and run across the street, run to your car, run to your office. Try to squeeze something like this in every day.

- Try dancing. It doesn't matter where—it can be in your bedroom, basement, or bathroom. Some of the songs I love to dance to are *Dancing Queen* by

ABBA (I am so ashamed to admit this!!!!), *Love Shack* by The B-52s, *Flashlight* by Parliament, *Planet Rock* by Afrika Bambaataa, *Staying Alive* by the BeeGees, and *Wipe Out* by the Fat Boys. When my youngest son was small we used to dance to songs like *Kung Foo Fighting* by Carl Douglas. As you can tell, I live in a crazy house, with a full and diverse iPod! Again, it is about moving and having fun by yourself or with your family.

• Take your sneakers on *every* vacation or trip. **Note:** *Be sure to keep sports-specific (e.g., walking, running, tennis, etc.) shoes that are well-fitting at all times. Also, be sure to replace them as they wear out. You can tell by the way they look or your feet / ankles / knees may start to hurt.* You have to fit exercise in, whether you are on vacation or not, but **especially** when you are eating more than usual. Who needs extra pounds added onto what you are already trying to lose? If you are not careful and proactive, vacations can get you into serious weight trouble. Believe me, I know! In fact I added this tip because of the foolishness I tend to indulge in during my summer vacations to Myrtle Beach, South Carolina. Myrtle Beach is a tradition for us. We absolutely love it!

However, every time we go, I literally lose my mind on the southern eating! We eat out for dinner ***EVERY*** night (my favorite place to eat is *Southern Suppers*, an all-you-can-eat restaurant that has such great food—fried flounder, fried shrimp, Polska Kielbasa sausage, turnip greens, corn bread muffins, and "sweet" tea!!!!), and I keep the fridge stocked with cookies and cream ice cream for the guys and chocolate ice cream bars for me. On the nights when they might leave me alone in the room while they go out to play volleyball and listen to music, I could eat at least four ice cream bars in a row! Each time I do this, I feel so ashamed!!!!!!! BUT THEY ARE SO GOOOOOD!!!!!! I have often hidden the empty boxes in the trash, and then I would go out and buy more the next day. Keep in mind that I am the main person eating them. I am also ashamed to admit that we even visit *Dairy Queen* and *Dipping Dots* while we are there!

I am sure none of you have ever indulged in this level of foolishness on your vacations, but when I go to Myrtle Beach, I just do not know how to eat like I have some sense after breakfast and lunch. It is just a fact of life! Be that as it may, my goal is to make sure that *what is done at Myrtle Beach stays at Myrtle Beach!* So I step up my activity level: my husband and I play tennis with the kids most days, I do a combination of jogging and walking most mornings, the boys and I play paddleball on the beach, I dance on the deck with my husband at night, I try to swim a couple of times, and I make sure we walk wherever we can as much as we can. This is why sneakers and workout gear are essential. So to keep yourself out of trouble, be sure to walk, run, swim, dance, *do whatever you must*, but try not to leave vacations with extra weight.

- Find ways to step up the physical activity as you go through periods where you are not as active as you should be. During colder months, I am not always consistently active, so I tend to make up reasons to go from the bottom level of my house to the top, to do jumping jacks and push-ups with my sons or have jump rope or hula hoop contests. The contests are the most fun, but they have become very strenuous because the boys are so competitive. However, that is one of the downsides/perks of working out with your kids.

- Based on the last suggestion, I would say if you have kids, you should definitely get them involved in more of your physical activities. One thing that my oldest son has said to me that has influenced me in this area and touched my heart was, "*I want you to take care of yourself so that you are healthy when you are older so you can still do things with us.*" That almost made me cry because "doing things" with my children is one of my life's greatest pleasures—I love to run, play, and laugh with them, especially when I can at least keep up with them. I promised my son I would do my best to take care of myself and try to stay as healthy as I can because it is my prayer that I am playing with their children's children one day. *Wouldn't that be a great blessing if we were all still active and at a healthy weight in our later years?* Well, the more we move today, the better chance we have of that happening in our future.

Some of the more fun activities that we have done include walking to a park with a baseball diamond, where we let the kids hit the ball while we work the field. I would make myself run a lot to get the ball, and my husband would pitch me a few so I could get a few runs in. Playing with kids—yours or someone else's (e.g., kickball, catch, touch football, etc.) is a win-win solution. *It is good for you and them.* Also, you are creating memories that will last a lifetime.

- If you plan to get exercise in after dinner, you should put your workout clothes on *before* you even start preparing dinner. By the time you eat, if you have to find an outfit, shoes, socks, *and* then get dressed, time will get away from you. You will get tired, something will come up, and you will lose the resolve you initially had to work out. However, if your clothes and shoes are already on, the battle to get exercise is already half way over.

There have been times where I was not dressed after dinner, but instead of looking for the perfect workout outfit, I just put on my sneakers and walked outside or got on the treadmill wearing what I was already wearing (e.g., jeans and a turtleneck, slacks and a blouse, casual dress, wool skirt, etc.). This may require me to take off a few layers while on the treadmill to the extent where my sons have come in only to say, "*Yuck*" because I am wearing a bra and jeans. Our treadmill is in a room in the basement, so I start off feeling cold, which makes me not want to work out at all. However, the comfort of a shirt/or turtleneck, the warmth of a space heater, a good book to read and a show on television are enough to help me get over my initial desire to bundle up with a blanket and watch television. After about fifteen minutes of fast-paced walking, the turtleneck/shirt is gone, and the space heater gets turned off. By then, I am sufficiently motivated to continue. Is this a little unorthodox? Of course it is, but it gets me off the couch. That's what this is all about, so get a little unorthodox if you must, but get moving!

- If you are more than twenty pounds overweight, I would not spend a lot of time doing sit-ups or buying machines to spot reduce (e.g., flatten your stomach, reduce your thighs, etc.). I think these types of exercises may be good once you are already on a path to losing weight. However, until you are, this type of focused attention could lead to bulkier muscle underneath the fat, which means you could have more noticeable bulges than you already do. Before you can have a flatter stomach or firmer legs, excess fat must be dealt with first. This means you have to move consistently, and as you will learn in the next chapter, *eat like you have some sense.* Whatever you can do to get your heart rate up to burn calories, do it. Until then, I would leave the infomercial machines and efforts to firm up alone until you can get your weight down. As I say this, please don't think I am advising you to avoid strength-training because I am not—*building muscle is definitely a good thing because muscle burns more calories than fat.* However, I think you should focus your efforts on the *get moving* part first, and then add other components as you are comfortable. Trust me, just to get moving consistently will be hard enough!

- For those of you who might be at a weight or a point where you are not able to do much physically, I completely understand if you are struggling to get started. *So with your doctor's permission…* I suggest you just start off by doing whatever physical activity you can. If that means just walking around the outside of your house once or twice a day, just do that. What about to your mail box or around the block? Only you know your limitations, but once you find out what you are capable of doing, *do whatever you can,* and add to it as you are able. Even if your eating habits stay the same, just increasing your activity level could stabilize your weight. So that is certainly better than nothing because it could at least keep your weight from spiraling out of control. Then, once you decide to be more active and get your eating under control, losing weight will be that much easier. So don't be discouraged if you have to start off with small steps.

I hope these suggestions have inspired you to get moving. *I simply cannot let you leave this chapter without being 100 percent sold on the idea that daily activity is absolutely essential for losing / maintaining your weight, as well as your physical, emotional, and mental well-being!* If you do, I have not done my job. In fact, I feel it is my mission to let you know that the more you move, the easier it gets, but it all starts with that first step. Even if you have never been active in your life, no matter your age, it is not too late, and YOU CAN DO IT! So let's agree that you will lose any defeatist attitude you may have (e.g., I can't commit to going to the gym, or I hate aerobics, so there is no point in exercising at all, etc.). Instead, try saying, I hate aerobics and going to the gym, but *I like to* _____ (e.g., walk, swim, play tennis, dance to my favorite songs, etc.). Or I can't run, but *I can* _____ (e.g., do jumping jacks, jump rope, play catch with my kids, throw a Frisbee with my kids/spouse, etc.). ***Being active must be more about what you can do*** and what you enjoy than it is about what you can't do. The goal is to just *start* SOMEWHERE.

Losing Baby-Weight

Now that I have hopefully sold you on the benefit of getting out and moving, I want to address another area of weight loss that can be very frustrating to deal with—the reality of coming home from the hospital after having a baby with twenty-five, thirty, or fifty plus pounds to lose. I don't know about you, but I just knew that most of the forty plus pounds I gained during my pregnancies would just melt away after the babies were born. *Not!* I think my hopes were also fueled by the stories of how breastfeeding just burns so many calories. Maybe it did, but obviously not enough to undo the damage I caused by having an eating-good-time while I was pregnant! In fact, during the first two months after the babies, I did not look anything like the woman I used to be, I was someone completely different. *I was actually someone's mother*, which was absolutely wonderful (*especially when you added in the two "bonuses" that were naturally augmented by milk*), but my weight was in the 170s! This part was not wonderful in any way, especially since the weight was determined not to go anywhere without a fight. *I had to really get serious before the scale started moving in the right direction.*

For the new, or even not so new, mothers that are trying to lose baby-weight, you are going to have to get serious where exercise is concerned if you want to get the scale moving in the right direction quickly. *Especially if you have quite a bit of weight to lose.* So to help you with that task, I'd like to share a mini-plan that I came up with just for this purpose. Quite honestly, it can be used by anyone who has a large amount of weight to lose, but I put it in this section because I used it specifically to battle "baby" fat. However, you can use it to lose weight, regardless of how it was gained...

As I've mentioned before, I think walking is always a great place to start, which is what I did. Even though both of my sons were born in November, I still took a few short walks in my neighborhood while they were sleeping. When weather permitted, I would bundle them up in their stroller and take them out for walks as well. However, the scale was not impressed by the walking I was doing. Finally, I had to accept the fact that I was going to have to do more than this if I wanted to be back in my size 6 clothes by spring. As a result, I asked for a treadmill for Christmas, and I *decided* that once the doctor gave me the green light for exercise, I was going to start some sort of plan. *I had no idea what that plan would be though…*

When I finally reached the six-week mark, and the doctor gave me the green light for strenuous exercise, I asked myself, "*What is the maximum I think I can do today?*" I wasn't sure since I wasn't in the best shape, but I thought I should at least be able to walk a mile. *Surely I could do that.* If I couldn't, I was in even worse shape than I thought! So that became my starting goal, and the plan became to slowly, but surely, increase my endurance on the treadmill. This included at least a mile of moderate walking (the first few minutes were set aside for a relatively slow warm-up and the last two for a cool down). I started off slowly, so it took me about twenty plus minutes, but this was something I could commit to at least five days a week.

So my first piece of advice to you? Figure out what "your" starting goal is: maybe it is a quarter or a half mile on the treadmill, a block or a few blocks of walking in your neighborhood, or a few times up the stairs in your house. It doesn't really matter where you start, *just as long as you start…* I walked that mile for about a week or so until I was comfortable doing it. As I got comfortable, I gradually walked a little faster, added arm movement, and even a gradual incline. The next step was to increase the amount of walking by a minute each time. As an example, if I walked twenty-three minutes, the next day I'd do twenty-four, and the next maybe twenty-five, or if I walked 1.1 miles one day, the next day I might push it to 1.2 miles. Even on days where I didn't increase the time or distance, I might just increase the incline earlier in the routine.

Over a three-month period, I went from walking one mile in twenty plus minutes to walking/running over three miles in a little under an hour. I have to admit the running really jump-started things. I got the idea from my husband who played college soccer, which requires you to run at top speeds during a ninety-minute game. To get in shape for the season, the team would go through intensive cardio routines (e.g., running until someone threw up, running up the bleachers in Death Valley's stadium, etc.). At that time, his thighs were chiseled, and he had a washboard stomach. He used to always tell me if I wanted to slim my midsection, I needed the up-and-down motion of running or fast-paced walking. Based on his advice, while the babies napped, I continued my combination of walking and running (I ran more and more as time progressed) on the treadmill five days a week, doing a little more each time. I also started adding mini-squats at the end of the routine, where I would pretend like I was sitting in a chair and hold that position for thirty seconds. In addition to this routine, I still took the kids for walks in their strollers during the week and on the weekends.

The point is to **push yourself a little more each time, as you are able**. If you are doing laps at a track, add running up the bleachers once or twice to the end of the routine. Or after you get off the treadmill, add jumping rope, floor work with a medicine/stability ball, and/or push-ups to your routine (*this is what I do—in fact, I jump rope two hundred plus times inspired by Michelle Obama and do crunches with a medicine or stability ball*). If you have been running up the stairs in your home, try to double your efforts in the course of a day, or add ten jumping jacks or push-ups (great for strength training and preventing bone loss) at the end of the routine. I think you get the idea—*the more you do, the faster you will see results, and the more dramatic those results will be*. Guess what else? The more you do, *the more you can do*, which is very exciting.

Another idea to try is to increase your intensity after you reach your goal distance (e.g., quarter mile, half mile, one mile, one set of stairs, etc.), you may want to alternate moderate walking with speed walking or light jogging—say walk five minutes, jog/speed walk one or two minutes. If you are taking stairs, you could just take them a little faster or take them a few more times a day. Also, if you walk one lap around a track, try running up the bleachers in between laps. If you walk one lap, maybe jog/run the other. I have heard that varying the intensity of your workout is a great thing to do because it supposedly burns more calories than walking or running at the same pace for the entire workout. Based on my experiences, I believe it.

As you add on to your routine, don't think that you can't add walks, stairs, or other activities in as you have time or as it makes sense. This is basically what

I meant when I suggested you create a lifestyle of movement. Can you believe that the simple walk/jog routine that I just shared, *combined with a lifestyle of movement*, got me back into my size 6 clothes after each baby? I even had a flat stomach *after a Cesarean delivery!* I was thrilled! A relative had once told me that after a Cesarean my stomach would never be flat again—*I am so glad she was wrong!* I don't know if it was the walking/running, the great surgical work of my ob/gyn at the time (*Dr. Andrea Jackson—she's the best*), or a mixture of both, but my stomach was flat without any sit-ups or abdominal work. So the advice I have shared really worked for me, and I never felt better in my life. Maybe a similar plan could work for you. I am sure it can, but, I must say yet again, before you get started on a plan like this, **check with your doctor first.** Once you get the green light, why not give it a try? *What do you have to lose but weight?* If you are medically and physically able to do it, and then you commit to it for at least three months, I know you won't be disappointed!

My Mini-Fitness Wake-Up Call

Regardless of your age, I am sure there have been times where you thought you were in pretty good shape, but then something put you to the test physically (e.g., you had to run to catch a bus/train/plane/child, you played a game against someone younger, etc.), and you had to face the fact that that you are nowhere close to being in the shape you thought you were. I am sure many of you can relate, but even if you can't, I certainly have! In fact, I had a mini wake-up call as I ran through an airport with my family to catch a plane that was on the final boarding call. I can't recall the airport, but it was one of the larger ones like in Atlanta, Georgia, where the gates are spread far apart. I was doing a mixture of running/jogging/speed-walking with my husband and sons well ahead of me. Although I was carrying my laptop and one of my son's backpacks, I could not believe how out of breath I was after only about five minutes. By the time we got close to the gate (less than a mile away), it felt like my heart was literally jumping out of my chest, and I was fighting to breathe.

Even though I was forty at the time, I knew this was not good, and *I was scared.* I started to think, "What if I had been running for my life?" *Would that have been as far, or as fast, as I could go?* If so, then I would have been in trouble! I probably would have given up like a lot of the girls usually do in horror movies such as *Friday the 13*[th] and *Halloween*. Funny, but not good. Add this to the fact that my chest felt weird as I breathed over the next few hours, I found myself saying yet again, "**I don't want to go out like this!**" *So what if I can wear the size clothes that I want and can look decent in them if I am not in good physical shape?* This episode helped me to see that it is not all about how you look, but more about the health of your body. I have to tell you, my body let me know real quick, "*Hey, you are not in the kind of shape you thought!*" I have to admit that I was very surprised because I took the stairs at work, played games with my sons and walked occasionally. *Obviously not enough.*

The only positive thing I could take away from this incident was the fact that I knew my heart was fine because I had recently had an EKG and blood work that concluded that my heart was fine, and I was not anemic. Also, I do not have asthma or any other type of breathing condition. So I thought I was in decent enough shape where I could run a short distance without feeling like I was having an asthma/heart attack! *Wrong!* Needless to say during our flight, I was concerned and sad about the little fitness test that I had just failed. I didn't share any of this with my family, but I felt that I was at a crossroad where my health and fitness were concerned. Isn't it is funny and symbolic that this would happen to me at forty? I think so, and at times such as these, when our bodies don't perform the way we might expect, we have two choices:

1) Say "*oh well*," and accept the fact that as we get older, we can't do the things we used to, and make it a point not to run like that again thinking our hearts can't take it (*basically accept this as your fate, and give up*); or
2) Take this as a sign that your heart needs more exercise, and do something about it.

As you might have guessed, I chose option two: **I decided to do something about it!** So during our vacation, we walked extensively *every day* (it helped that we were in Orlando visiting *Disney* and that there were restaurants we could walk to for dinner), we rode bikes at our resort, and we ran/walked around a jogging path during most days. You notice I said "*we*." As I mentioned before, whenever possible, getting in shape should be a family affair. When we came home, after eating way too much junk, we jogged to the boys' school and played kickball against them. Again, my body was saying, "*What are you doing?*" The next day I went to the gym for the first time after a year, and I worked out and loved it. Afterward, I did some work on this book as I watched my sons swim.

During our second jogging session, I was praying just to make it to the light that is about a quarter of a mile from our house! By the third or fourth time we did it, I was surprised that I continued jogging while I waited for the light to change, and I was finally able to make it up the hill and continue running. Even though I was winded, I surprised myself by making it all the way to the school (it really helps to have goal when you are working out). We played kickball once we got there, and I can't tell you how much I was huffin' and puffin' afterward, but on the way home after walking a block or so I felt like jogging again. That was kind of odd, but I said maybe I can just jog back the first block, but then next thing you know, I had jogged almost all of the way home—with my oldest son running behind me, instead of in front as he had been. He was shocked and impressed, and *so was I*. Guess what else? My chest didn't hurt, and I could breathe easily... After a while I realized, "Hey this isn't as terrible as I thought—*I might actually like to run*." Maybe a little—*certainly not a lot*.

A few days later I was actually looking forward to exercising with my family that evening. Strange, but true. *However,* when I got home, the kitchen needed to be cleaned, dinner needed to be cooked, kids had homework to be checked... I was hungry and tired... I wanted to run, but it was almost 7:00... My youngest son had itchy/red eyes from the massive tree pollen... He did not need to be outside... *I was no longer motivated*... All of a sudden, I just wanted to get in the bed, eat cake, watch *24* and *The Apprentice*, and do a little work in the kitchen and on my laptop... However, my oldest son said, "*Mom, are you ready to go running and play basketball?*" I wanted to say no, but instead I said, "*Yes, go put your shoes on...*"

I let him know that we weren't going to play long or go far because it was so late... We ran to the court, and although my heart was beating like crazy, we played a short game of full court basketball. For once in years, I won (I think he took it easy on me). Finally a few kids his own age came, and while they played, I jogged around the court. At first, I thought I would do it five times, but then I decided to try ten, then fifteen, and then twenty. I was shocked at how much I could do. Afterward, I felt more energized to go home and tackle the homework, dinner, and dishes that were waiting for me—*of course, they were still there*. However, my son and I had spent some quality time together, we both got much-needed exercise, and my fitness level was being restored to where it needed to be. So what are the takeaway lessons? **Don't accept what you see today as your unchangeable fate.** Involve your family and friends as much as possible in your quest to get/stay in shape, and the more you can do exercise-wise, the better!

<u>Going the Extra Mile</u>

Surely by now you have many examples of what you can do to get out and get moving. I don't want you to ever be limited to just one means of activity or exercise because that makes the whole process boring and reduces your chances of long-term success. Believe me, there are so many opportunities in our everyday lives where we can incorporate exercise. In fact, one of the things I have not mentioned is the fact that I also have a little routine that I do most mornings before I get out of bed. So you can even start exercising before you are fully awake! I don't do much, but the little routine actually helps me to wake up.

All I do is hold my ankles or touch my toes as my feet face the ceiling for thirty seconds. Then I lower my legs and raise them and my torso/arms to make a 45-degree angle. I hold this position for thirty seconds (my body is in a "V" shape). I do both moves twice, and then I lay flat. Next, I bend one knee and touch it to the opposite side of the bed and hold. I do the same thing for the other knee. Then on the way to the bathroom, I do push-ups (the kind men do, I can do twenty at a time—they are really good for your stomach as well as your arms). I come out of the push-up position by inching my hands back toward my feet until I am in an upside down "V" with my hands as close to being palm down as they can. I hold this stretch position for thirty seconds as well (no bouncing though). Even though I think it is extremely important for us to be very active from a cardiovascular standpoint, I still think we have to remember to keep strength straining and stretching in the picture in order to prevent bone loss and shortening ligaments, which can lead to inflexibility and unnecessary injuries as we age. *None of us need or want that.* To finish my morning routine, I also do leg lifts (side and back), as well as mini-squats while I am brushing my teeth. *Every little bit helps!*

Make Your Move

As I said, my main exercise is walking (*even when my knee hurts*), usually fast paced in my neighborhood, but the treadmill is my backup and supplement. A few months ago, I bought the *Walk-Vest* to wear while I am on the treadmill. It is a weighted vest that Valerie Bertinelli said she wore to enhance her walking workouts, so I ordered one from *Amazon.com*. I had the thought that I would wear it outside, but my sons said I looked ridiculous, so I just wear it on the treadmill. Does it work? *Who knows, but it certainly can't hurt!* Also, as I am mentioning the treadmill, I was wondering... Do you think I actually enjoy using it? Well to be honest, it can be kinda boring, and it feels like work. So the answer is no. However, I can get myself to do at least forty-five minutes if I watch a show/ movie or read a book that feels really self-indulgent such as a Harlequin Romance book. Even though I enjoy reading on the treadmill, I will admit that it is not the safest thing to do. In fact, I tried it at the gym on one of the treadmills that has a rough surface, and I stumbled a couple of times. I have never had a problem on smooth surfaces though. Be that as it may, I can't advise anyone to do this, but if you do it, **please be careful!** I should also mention that I only read if I am walking (no running/jogging).

Even though I mentioned that I don't like to go to the gym, I still go occasionally on the weekend if it is raining and my sons want to play basketball. My gym routine includes: stretching on the mat, which consists of me touching my toes in a number of different ways and holding it for a count of thirty seconds; thirty-forty minutes on an elliptical machine (I especially like the ones that are hands-free because I can read); fifteen minutes of fast-paced walking on the treadmill and then more stretching on the mat to further loosen my warmed-up muscles. On the days where I have already walked in my neighborhood before coming, my husband and I might just shoot around or play a few games of basketball with our boys. None of these activities are complicated or intensive, but they all help keep me where I want to be—*able to run at least a mile if I need to so I am not back at the point I was in my mini-fitness wake-up call.*

Speaking of that, I was at another airport more recently and getting ready to miss yet another connecting flight due to a delay. This time I was alone and wearing heels, but guess what? I ran as fast as those heels would allow for almost a mile. Of course I was a little winded and sweating, but I made it to the gate in time, and by the time I got on the plane, I was laughing and joking, and my heart was beating normally. Mission accomplished! *This is what I am talking about!* I want our bodies to be healthy enough and in shape enough to roll with life's punches as they come.

So the lesson I have learned/keep relearning, and that I am trying to share with you, is that we just have to *get moving, set goals,* and try to *stick with them.* Just doing this will revolutionize your activity level. Your routine does not have to be structured or formal, but **you do have to get moving**, and **you do need to work up a sweat as often as you can** (*at least thirty minutes a day is ideal*). Not only will your heart and waistline reap the benefits, but you will look better/younger and hopefully live a longer, healthier life. *That is my prayer for you.* However, it starts with you. So make your move today!

⌒

Chapter 8

Redefine & Reshape
Your Eating Habits
(Step 6)

Now that you have a better idea of where you are physically *and* where you need or want to be, *it is time for the main event*—the point where you turn your attention to your eating habits. I know it took a while to get all of the preliminary steps out of the way, but believe me, they are necessary if you are going to successfully change the habits of a lifetime. It is definitely a big undertaking, but well worthwhile. Changing your eating habits can literally *change* your life—*how you look, how you feel and your overall quality of life...* For this reason, I will spend a great deal of time in this chapter getting you to *redefine* and *reshape* your eating habits.

I am sure you must be asking, *"How on earth, do we do that?"* Well, I tell you it is not easy to do when we live in a society where food is constantly being pushed at us left and right as we go about our daily lives. However, *it can be done*, and it becomes easier and easier as you learn to make better food choices. *Why does everything always boil down to choices?* The old saying is definitely true: *choices are long-lasting and life-changing.* So making better food choices must be a priority if we are going to have a healthy weight for life. That's where my lifestyle methodology of *Eating Like You Have Some Sense* comes in... So the next few sections will exhaustively cover:

• Learning To Eat Like You Have Some Sense
• Eating Like You Have Some Sense

A lot of information will be given for both sections, but all it really boils down to is helping you modify your everyday eating habits so you can enjoy your favorite foods while losing and/or maintaining your weight. In the past your relationship with food may have been complicated—going back and forth between love and hate, but this chapter should help change that. I want to help you *redefine* your relationship with food—*so that you eat it to live, not live to eat it.* I also hope to help *reshape* your habits by giving you ideas you never thought of to help you *moderately* eat the foods you enjoy as if you have some sense. Once you are doing this consistently, you will be well on your way to a healthy weight for life! In the meantime, let's start off by learning to *eat like we have some sense...*

ᘒ

Learning To Eat
Like You Have Some Sense
~ . ~ . ~ ~ . ~ . ~ . ~

I know I have made you wait forever to get to the heart and soul of the book, and I am sorry, but I don't think the advice in this chapter can be successfully applied until all of the other *stuff* has been dealt with... I mean you have to know what is *eating* you, and deal with it (*I hope you have*). Your mind must be right (*I hope it is*). You have to know exactly where you are and be ready to make a commitment to change (*I hope you are*). You also need a plan/idea on how you will consistently get moving (*I hope you do*). Have you honestly considered all of these areas? If you have, I think you are ready to move forward. However, if you haven't, you may need to revisit some of the areas that you might have struggled with so you are sure that you are *really* ready to get started. I say this because there are so many factors that drive the way we eat that if we try to tackle the eating part without dealing with those issues first, you could be back at this same point within a matter of months. *That is not what I want for you.* **I want this to be the time that you achieve your weight loss goals once and for all.**

One of the issues I have had with other weight loss books over the years is that many just focus on eating right and exercising without addressing the issues that may cause us to overeat: untreated medical conditions (e.g., anemia, thyroid conditions, etc.); stress; emotional baggage; a life that is out of balance; a life that does not include work/activities that make us happy or fulfilled; messages and social cues from the food and advertising industries (e.g., portion sizes have doubled so we have adjusted our perception of what a meal/snack should be); etc. The forces that drive us to overeat are complicated, so I want us to treat them as such. If we don't, long-lasting success will be elusive, if not downright impossible. This is why I don't think diets work... Most of them don't acknowledge that we are overeating for reasons other than hunger (e.g., trying to fill a void, not happy with the way our lives are going, feeling out of control, etc.).

What Brought Us to This Low?

When I go out to restaurants, movie theaters, and amusement parks, I often look around to see what people are eating and drinking, and based on what I see I am convinced that many of us are *eating ourselves to death*, or at least sick. The evidence is showing as our weight, *and the weight of our kids*, is spiraling out of control. This is the heaviest we have been as a country, and the rates of type 2 diabetes, hypertension, and heart disease are increasing right along with our weight. Don't get me wrong; it is OK to indulge occasionally, but we have gone *way* beyond the occasional indulgence. We are doing it week in and week out, and we have got to stop it if we want to live the rich, productive lives God intended us to have. So as I look at where we are and try to figure out how to get us back on track, I think it makes sense to ask the question what brought us to this low? To be fair, we, as consumers, did have help in getting where we are with our eating habits.

I find the relationship between restaurant owners/advertisers and consumers almost like the one between the chicken and the egg—which came first: the introduction of "*Hey Kool-Aid*" and "*Have a Coke and a smile*" commercials *or* our desire to drink less water? The removal of green vegetables and fruits from most restaurant menus *or* our desire to eat fries or baked potatoes with meals instead? The introduction of larger food servings in restaurants *or* our desire to eat more at one sitting? I could be wrong, but I am thinking that businesses decided to capitalize on our greed, and like some sort of pusher they keep thinking of more and more ways to keep us coming back. Vanilla ice cream is no longer enough, we have to have it with *Oreos*, cookie dough, cheesecake, or pieces of candy bars mixed in it now. Plain strawberry, vanilla, or chocolate shakes are no longer enough, we now have all sorts of ingredients added in to make what used to be a naughty little indulgence into a massive overindulgence that has enough calories and fat for two or three meals! Don't get me wrong; we are ultimately responsible for what we buy and eat, but I don't think we wound up at this point all by ourselves—*WE DEFINITELY HAD HELP!*

I have to tell you I get really upset when I see the serving sizes for adults and children today. Most restaurants give enough fries in their kids' entrees to feed two or three adults! Also, many restaurants have done away with kid-sized hamburgers, so they give kids an adult-sized version. Am I the only one who is alarmed by this? I don't think a ten- or eleven-year-old needs an adult-sized burger, two or three servings of fries in one, and a soda that comes with free refills. However, because we have gotten so used to seeing this almost everywhere we go, we have come to accept this as a "normal," acceptable meal for kids or even ourselves. Then we wonder why we are gaining weight as we continue to eat like this. I almost feel like we have been subjected to some sort of commercial brainwashing, and I feel fortunate to have woken up in time. So now when I go to one of my favorite restaurants for a barbeque pork sandwich, even though the plate is piled high with mouth-watering fries, I have enough resolve to eat only a few or none at all. I have started asking the waiter not to even bring them. This is because after having the crispy crust of the rolls (*I don't like the inside*) and half of an appetizer, I am almost full. So I take half (or more) of the sandwich home. I drink water, and I don't even look at the dessert menu. *I am no longer brainwashed and addicted, but this was not always the case...*

Eating Like *I* Didn't Have Any Sense

Growing up, I was a troubled and lonely teenager who desperately wanted to be slim. However, I remember being able to eat a *Big Mac*, large fries, and soda around 3:30, and by 5:00 I was ready to eat a banana split from *Dairy Queen*. Afterward, I might take a nap, and I would be ready to eat dinner by 7:00! So as we already covered in Chapter 4, there was obviously something *eating* me (e.g., absentee father, sexual molestation, etc.); otherwise, I would not have been eating so much unless I was running ten to fifteen miles every day or had a tapeworm! So on one hand I wanted to be slim, but I couldn't eat like I had some sense to save my life! I think most of the problem was emotional, but another component was the fact that no one ever talked to me about not eating any and everything that I wanted, whenever I wanted to. Of course I knew that I should not eat junk or drink sweet drinks right before dinner because it could spoil my appetite, but beyond that, I ate whatever I wanted, *whenever I wanted.* No one told me to drink water, no one reminded me to eat fruit instead of junk. No one ever talked to me about the consequences of overeating or snacking constantly. I can't remember a time where an adult asked, *"Why are you eating that snack, didn't you just have some cookies and a soda?"* My eating knew no boundaries, especially when I went to college.

As I mentioned before, college was a very stressful place for me, and I seriously struggled with my weight there. Things could have been so much worse, but for me, it was as bad as I ever wanted it to get. I remember desperately wanting to shop in a store called 5-7-9 (the name reflected the sizes of the clothes they sold), but at the time it seemed like an impossible dream. I guess I could blame it on the *freshman fifteen*, even though I was no longer a freshman, and I couldn't fit the sizes in that store even before I went to college! To make matters worse, one of my slimmer friends commented that she did not know how to describe me. She said she would not call me fat, but she would not call me slim either. Maybe she was looking for the word "chunky"—either way, I wished she had kept her thoughts to herself, *but she didn't.* My feelings were obviously hurt then because I still remember the comment today…

However, the "chunky" label should have been understandable when I look back at how I was eating… For breakfast I would head to the cafeteria most mornings and get grits, bacon, eggs, sausage, fruit, and juice. Sometimes they might even have doughnuts, which I would have with cereal, milk, and fruit. For a late morning snack I would often grab a candy bar or chips. For lunch I would head back to the cafeteria for my usual breaded chicken patty, fries, fruit, soda, and maybe a cookie or two (*I was not used to having so many choices*). After my classes, I would take a nap and/or go to the campus store to get a sixteen-ounce soda and a large pack of cookies or a candy bar. Otherwise, I would snack in my room, drinking soda from a two-liter bottle and eating chips or cookies from a bag (*Oreos* and *Chips Ahoy* were my favorite). Two hours later, I would go back to the cafeteria for dinner: usually a burger or something fried (e.g., chicken, fish, shrimp, etc.) and fries, with vegetables tossed in for good measure. I drank soda or sweet tea with my meals during this time—*never water*. For dessert, I usually had ice cream, cookies, or cake. I wish I could say that this was all I would eat in a day, but I would still enjoy a number of other snacks in the evening. Basically, I had an eating good time!

Looking back, I think the meal plan was almost a license for me to eat like I didn't have any sense—unlimited food, snacks, and drinks were at my fingertips for breakfast, lunch, and dinner. However, there was a time when I modified my meal plan to save money so it just included breakfast and lunch. Even though I was *supposed* to be saving money, I would often order a pizza with a two-liter soda, or I would get one of my favorite meals from *Bojangles*: a steak and egg biscuit, a sausage and egg biscuit, AND a drumstick. Oh yeah, I forgot, I would also have soda! If I didn't eat one of these *well-balanced* meals, I would get a twelve-inch steak and cheese sub and chips with a soda. You would think that would be more than enough food for the day, but I also ate and drank throughout the night as I studied. I don't think I saved any money with this revised meal plan. In fact, I probably wound up spending and eating more! Could I really have been this hungry? *No, of course not.*

I believe I was trapped in a cycle of emotional eating, and I was constantly thinking about what I was going to eat next. Can you say *self-medicating?* Looking back at how I used to eat provides a wonderful example of eating like you *don't* have any sense. However, to come to my defense, I just never learned any better, and the commercials on television made it all look so normal. Remember the ads about *how you can't eat just one?* Well, *I couldn't.* There had never been any checks and balances placed on my eating before, and there certainly weren't any in college. In fact, this was a time in my life where I didn't have much else going on other than school; there was no boyfriend, very few close friends, and even fewer close family ties. Food had become my recreation/companion/*drug of choice*, and a big part of my life was looking forward to what I was going to eat next. If I was going to be in for the weekend with nothing to do, I would always have a food(s) in mind that I planned to eat (e.g., cookies, candy bars, *Hot Fries*, etc.), and there would usually be a two-liter bottle of soda to go with it. This all felt very normal then, but *this style of eating should never be the norm.*

Eating Like We *Don't* Have Any Sense

As I am sure you would agree, I ate a lot back then, but do you think I was well-nourished? No, in fact, I was chronically anemic to the point I couldn't even give blood without fainting. A lot of times we think because we eat so much that we are healthy, but that is not necessarily the case. A few years ago I remember reading about a man who weighed over four hundred pounds, but he was not healthy enough to have surgery because of severe malnutrition. I am sure he was just as shocked to hear it as I was to read it, but maybe we shouldn't be shocked at all… When you think about it, many of us are eating a lot, but much of it is junk. The term junk-food is definitely appropriate because it accurately describes what we are consuming on a regular basis—foods and drinks with little or no nutritional value.

I honestly believe many of us are eating ourselves to death. We eat too much meat, processed foods and sweets, and we drink way too much soda, coffee, and alcohol. We were meant to eat fruits, vegetables, and whole grains and to drink water on a *daily* basis. Raise your hand if days go by, and you don't remember if you have had any of these items. Don't feel too bad if your hand is up, because you are not alone. However, if we don't find a way to change this, our futures won't be as healthy and bright as they should be. How did our eating get so out of control anyway? I think it could be due to the fact that those of us living in the most developed countries have bought into the convenience of fast-food, have become hooked on sugar-laden treats, eat larger portions, and we often eat like television-controlled zombies. Commercials used to just tempt us, but now they are shaping *how*, *when,* and *what* we eat and drink. We are out of control, and *we are literally eating like we don't have any sense.* I know that may be harsh, but it is true, and I am not just talking to you, but to myself as well.

What do I mean by "eating like we don't have any sense"? Well, for one thing this may mean that we are "living to eat" instead of *eating to live*, which means there is a constant preoccupation with eating. For example, if you go to the mall, is your first thought *Auntie Anne's* or *Cold Stone Creamery* even if you have already eaten? For kids, I can understand their strong desire to eat every treat they see, but for mature adults, we should be able to walk on by in most cases. Another example is if you are going to the movies, is your first thought a large popcorn with butter, the largest soda they have and a pretzel or a box of candy even if you have already eaten a full dinner? Again, kids may not know any better, but for those of us who do this on a regular basis, it may be an indicator that we are living to eat or eating like we don't have any sense. Fortunately we can enjoy these types of indulgences *occasionally* without major repercussions in our health or weight. However, if you find yourself *continually* overindulging in high-fat, high-calorie treats/foods, **and** you are struggling with your weight, changes may be needed. Examples of some of these hurtful habits include:

1. Visiting vending machines or fast-food restaurants for breakfast more than once or twice a week.
2. Visiting vending machines more than three or four times a week for snacks.
3. Eating frozen entrees more than three or four times a week.
4. Eating meals with processed foods more than once or twice a week (e.g., hot dogs, *Spam*, *Steak-Ums*, bacon, sausage, *Ramen Noodles*, etc.).
5. Eating fries more than once or twice a week.
6. Eating more than one meal a day that doesn't include fruits or vegetables.
7. Having bread, an appetizer, dinner (especially if it includes fries), drinks, **and** dessert at restaurants on a regular basis.
8. Eating at restaurants more than once a day when you are not traveling or on vacation.
9. Eating out more than three or four times a week.
10. Drinking more than thirty-two ounces of soda a week (*diet or regular*).
11. Drinking more than one alcoholic beverage a day.

12. Eating more than one large bag of chips by yourself in a week.
13. Eating more than one large pack of cookies by yourself in a week.
14. Eating more than one large container of ice cream by yourself in a week.
15. Going to the store, or sending someone, more than once/twice a week for snacks.
16. Eating more than three large meals a day. *Remember, there is no fourth meal!*
17. Skipping lunch or dinner and eating junk instead on a regular basis.
18. Eating past the point of being full during meals.
19. Eating when you should be sleeping.
20. Eating meals in secret—you know, the ones you would be embarrassed for anyone to see you eat.
21. Eating meals, mainly fast-food, in your car.

Everyone has a weakness, and having one weakness is not as much of a problem, but if you are engaging in more than one or two of these activities on a regular basis, you may be eating and drinking like you don't have any sense. Obviously it is not an exact science; nor is this an exhaustive list. But in your heart of hearts, *you know if you have a problem*, and you know where it is, if you are honest with yourself. I have to admit I struggle to control myself in a couple of these areas, but let's face it, we will never be perfect. We are just setting general guidelines to keep our eating in check. Our weight and our overall health are good indicators of how well we are following these guidelines. I think sometimes changing our habits can be as simple as looking in the mirror and searching our hearts to get the confirmation we need to act.

How Do *You* Eat Like *You* Have Some Sense?

Now that I have told you so much about what you already know: *how bad our diets are, how badly we need to change our eating habits,* yadda, yadda, yadda, I am sure you are more than ready for me to tell you something that you don't already know. Well, I would be more than happy to do just that. Did you know that eating like you have some sense and maintaining a healthy weight in our gluttonous and stressed-out culture is still entirely possible and may be even easier than you think? The only catch is that you may have to tune out some of the information that is coming to you in the form of popular diet advice to do it. I know some diet experts and doctors are saying, *"Don't eat carbs, don't eat white flour, stay away from sugar, avoid dairy, etc.,"* but I will never agree with such blanket statements about our eating.

I really don't believe the average person can, or even has to, live within such rigid boundaries to be healthy and at a healthy weight. In fact, I bet you know people who have lived long, healthy lives eating all of the things we are supposed to be avoiding. I know I do, so I have to tell you this type of advice really gets on my nerves, and I want to ask: *Why can't we have carbs? Don't we need carbs to produce energy? Why can't we eat dairy products—don't we need the calcium!* Besides, regardless of what anyone says, I love milk, and **I am never giving it up!** *Also, why can't we have any sugar?* Are all of the studies really in on these artificial sweeteners (e.g., *Splenda, Equal,* etc.)??? I have to tell you, I am very skeptical about their use. In fact, I limit my kids' intake of products containing these sweeteners mainly because I have gotten a headache or a queasy feeling every time I ate or drank products containing them. I know some of you may like and trust them, but if you prefer sugar like me, wouldn't it be better to just eat the foods containing it in moderation instead of depriving ourselves?

I believe so. In fact, when we are constantly told, *"You can't have this"* or *"You can't have that,"* it creates an internal rebellion, and as is the case with children, we may "act out"—eating everything in sight/bingeing or yo-yo dieting, etc. None of this is good, and it won't help us reach or *maintain* a healthy weight, which should be our goal—*not just to reach that weight for a prom, wedding, trip, or a reunion, but for a lifetime.* That is the goal of this book, and this chapter is going to help you do just that by sharing tips and ideas to show you how to eat what you want in moderation. **Trade-offs and compromises will be necessary**, but I will never tell you what you "have to" eat or what you cannot eat.

To be successful for the long-term, I have found that you need to learn to eat foods that you are accustomed to eating *in moderation*, and build a healthy diet around that. This is key because *how* you eat to lose the weight is *how* you will have to eat for the long-term to keep the weight off. This is why I discourage the use of diet programs that *tell/sell* you what you have to eat. Think about it, what happens when you go back to eating "regular food" (*things you actually enjoy*) again? Your weight usually goes back to where it was before. This is why you must learn to *eat what you like* in moderation, *like you have some sense*. Otherwise, you will be stuck in an endless cycle of yo-yo dieting or always looking for the next great diet.

Say Good-bye to Diets Forever!

As I said before, I don't believe in diets, and I think most diet programs are a complete waste of time. Do you know why I feel so strongly? Well, for starters: I don't think they work for the long-term (*look around if you need proof*); they don't provide a solution or a cure, but more of a short-term fix or a Band-Aid; I think they make us think too much about the act of eating and take the fun out of it (I don't want to measure my chicken or know how many calories are in it); they make us dependent on someone else to tell us what/how to eat; and **they are expensive**! A few years ago, I read on *AOL* (under Money & Finance, in *Most Expensive Diets,* September 6, 2006) that the average American spends $54.50 per week on food; whereas the weekly diet for *Jenny Craig* costs $137.65. The article also stated that weekly diet costs for *Nutrisystem* were $113.52, for *Atkins* it was $100.52, for *Weight Watchers* it was $96.64, and for *Zone* it was $92.84. These figures are just for one person! I can't believe that people would spend almost double the money they are already spending on groceries *so* they can eat less food! *So let me get this straight, these programs are getting us to spend more money on food so we can eat less…* Does this make sense? I don't think so!

To be perfectly fair, I must admit that I have not verified these costs because I have never used or looked into these diets. However, I did find the *AOL* data interesting because it confirmed my suspicions about how pricey these plans *can* be. While I think the price should be a problem for most, I think the biggest problem with these programs is the dependence they can create among dieters, *as well as some of the payment plans dieters wind up with long after the food is gone.* Having food choices already made for us can keep us from ever learning how to eat moderately on our own, where we don't need food from a program. I believe this sets us up for failure. Say you do lose a significant amount of weight (e.g., ten pounds or more), how are you going to keep the weight off for the long-term if you stop eating the pre-packaged meals these companies sell? What happens when you go back to eating the way you did before you started the program? I'll tell you what will happen—*the weight will come right back!* This is why you hear of people going back to these programs every few years—because the weight usually comes back as soon as you start eating regular food (*food that **you** buy from the grocery store and prepare **yourself***).

So here's the bottom line: *until we learn how to eat the foods and drink the drinks that we can make or normally have access to, in moderation (like we have some sense), we won't have much success with long-term weight loss and maintenance.* Would you believe that losing and maintaining a healthy weight is really more about choices than it is about food (e.g., *Will I eat cereal for breakfast or doughnuts? Will I eat a banana while I wait for lunch or a Snicker's bar? Will I have a twenty-four-ounce soda with lunch or a glass of water? Will I eat a large bag of Doritos before dinner or a handful of walnuts and raisins?* etc.)? Believe it or not, the food and drink choices we make over time can help determine our weight more effectively than any diet program ever could. *The choice really lies within us.* So all you have to do now is *choose* to modify your existing eating habits so you can make the best choices as to *what* you put in your mouth and *when. Are you really ready to do this?* I surely hope you are because this type of behavior modification can change your life and your weight. To get the ball rolling, I have come up with another What-if model that can get you started:

What If...

1. You switched from whole milk to 2 percent milk? Drinking 1 percent or skim would be even better.
2. You switched to 2 percent or non-fat cheese in recipes and on sandwiches as often as you can?
3. You switched from regular white bread to whole-wheat bread? It would be even better if you tried the low-calorie variety. Either way the extra fiber will fill you up faster.
4. You ate cereal or oatmeal with low-fat milk for breakfast at least four/ five times a week?

5. You cut the amount of juice you drink by half, especially if you drink a lot? Also, make sure you are drinking 100 percent fruit juices, not juice cocktails that have added sugar.

6. You substituted an apple, orange, or banana for one of the snacks you eat each day?

7. You brought lunch/sandwich fixings (e.g., bread, lean deli meat, mustard, etc.) with you to work at least three times a week so you won't be as tempted to eat out?

8. You asked for only half the meat on your sub/sandwich at lunch? I bet you won't notice the difference—*my youngest son doesn't.*

9. You scooped out the excess bread on the inside of buns and sub bread? You won't be able to taste the difference, and you might save a few calories.

10. You used a napkin to dab excess grease off of your pizza and scooped any extra dough from under the toppings (pan pizza usually has a lot of extra dough between the topping and the crispy bottom)?

11. You squeezed your fried chicken between napkins to remove the excess grease before eating it? Although it can be messy, I have been doing this for years to make fried chicken a *little* healthier.

12. You used mustard, vinegar or seasonings (e.g., oregano, pepper, Italian seasonings, etc.) on subs and sandwiches instead of mayonnaise?

13. You added a little dressing at a time to your salads using your fork instead of plopping a big blob of it on the top? *Only use the minimum amount needed for taste.*

14. You substituted a can of vegetable soup or a couple of pieces of fruit for chips or fries as a side dish with your sub/sandwich/fried chicken/steak?

15. You ate a spicy pickle spear (I like the ones with garlic) instead of chips to satisfy your craving for salt? This is what I have started eating with my peanut butter and jelly sandwiches. You may not be better off from a sodium perspective, but you will save on fat and calories.

16. You kept fruit at your desk at work instead of going to a vending machine for snacks?

17. You cooked your own dinner at least four/five nights a week so you are eating in most of the week? The food you cook will have less fat/sodium, and you will tend to eat a lot less.

18. You didn't eat bread and butter at restaurants, especially if you are having an appetizer, fries with your meal, or dessert? You don't need all of these things in one sitting, do you?

19. You said no to appetizers and/or big, fancy drinks if you know you are having dessert?

20. You cut your entrée in half at restaurants and boxed up the other half to take home for dinner or tomorrow's lunch? **Not for a late-night snack though.**

21. You drank just one glass of soda at a restaurant, and when the server offered you a refill, you asked for water instead? A better choice would be just to drink water instead of soda, but if you *really, really* must have the soda, why not just have one?

22. You bought a large, insulated mug and kept it filled with ice water so you can sip during the day and night? *You will not be as hungry as often, trust me.*

23. You got rid of all of the foods in your house that you have no control over (*for me that would be Oreos, Keebler Fudge Covered Graham Crackers, Edy's Cookies & Cream ice cream, etc.*)? If you crave *Doritos* or *Cheetos*, enjoy a small bag, but don't bring home larger quantities than you *should* consume in one sitting. Enjoy a serving of ice cream at a store/stand, but don't bring home a carton if you know you cannot be trusted. This does not have to deprive your family—there are things that my family likes that I *can* be trusted with (e.g., non-chocolate candy, *YooHoo*, sugar/butter cookies, salt & vinegar potato chips, cookie dough ice cream, etc.). These things can be in the house forever, and I won't touch them. Everyone has a weakness—*find yours, and get it out of the house.*

24. You just ignored late-night stomach rumbling and drank some water, milk, tea, cocoa, or a small cup of juice (e.g., grape, pomegranate, orange, acai, prune, etc.) and went back to sleep? Unless you have just worked the late shift, you should not be eating late at night. *Believe me you won't starve before the morning.* Like I used to tell my husband, "You'll live—now go back to bed!"

25. You traveled with healthy food alternatives (e.g., fruit, low-fat bread and sandwich fixings, frozen water bottles, nuts, etc.) so you won't be

as tempted to reach for fast-food or other unhealthy choices that may be offered to you?

What do you think? Aren't there at least a few of these ideas you could implement today? *I bet there are.* So you now have a number of ideas on what you can do to start making relatively painless choices that can add up to major differences in your weight over time. However, there are a few other helpful questions I would like you to ask yourself:

1. Do you really need butter or margarine on the pancakes or waffles you are eating, or can you get by with just syrup?
2. Do you really need butter or margarine on your toast/croissant/biscuit, or can you get by with just jelly or preserves?
3. Can you live with syrup that has half the sugar of regular syrup (the lite varieties)?
4. Do you *really* have to cook food (e.g., eggs, omelets, grilled cheese, etc.) in butter, margarine, or shortening? Couldn't you use a non-stick spray such as *Pam* instead?
5. Do you really *have* to have sour cream, guacamole, and/or chili on your nachos, or can you get by with just salsa? Do you even need an appetizer *every* time you eat out?
6. If you put meat in your spaghetti sauce, can you cut the meat you use in half? I bet you won't even be able to taste the difference, but you will definitely cut calories/fat.
7. Instead of frying chicken or pork chops, couldn't you just bake or barbeque them?
8. Do you really need ice cream on your pie or cake?
9. Can you live with lite beer instead of regular, or just cut what you drink by half?
10. Would it *really* kill you to add a few more servings of fruits and vegetables to your diet?
11. If you stop at *McDonald's* for breakfast, can you live with just one *McGriddle* instead of two? Also, do you *really* need hash browns and a sausage patty to go with the hotcakes?

12. Would it *really* kill you to drink water with lunch and dinner, instead of soda or some other sweetened drink?
13. Do you *really* need a cappuccino, Frappuccino, or latte *every* day?
14. Do you *really, really* need to eat all of the fries that come with your meal *every* time? Are you really that hungry *every* time? Really think about this one.
15. Are you *really hungry* enough for seconds or thirds *every time* you eat? *Are you???*
16. Do you really need that late-night snack *every* night?

These questions are obviously not one-size-fits-all, but they may touch on areas that you might be struggling in—only you know what your areas of weakness are. However, if you know that there is something you can live without—*live without it.* If there are areas where you know you can do something differently—*do it.* If there is something you know you should stop doing—*stop it!* The first step to eating like you have some sense is doing what you know to do as often as you can. However, it is important that you remember as you go forward, if you choose unwisely or fall off the wagon for a day, week, month, or longer, *you have not failed.* You just need to work to get back on track as soon as you can, and keep reminding yourself that reaching your ideal weight and/or maintaining it is a lifelong journey that will have many ups and downs. So with that in mind, let's just try to make as many healthy choices as we can when we can, and keep our eye on the prize—*a healthier, slimmer body.*

Create an Environment Geared for Success

There are still a few more areas that must be addressed if you are going to succeed at eating like you have some sense. You have to make eating smarter and healthier a family affair. I am not saying that the whole family has to restrict their eating, but healthier food choices that everyone can enjoy should be available at all times. Unfortunately all children and spouses are not the same, so the *food manager* of the family (usually the mom) has to consider the likes/dislikes of the family members at a high level. Let's face it, the happier your family is with their food choices, the more likely they will be to support you and eat like they have some sense. So before I stopped buying things like chocolate chip cookies, *Oreos,*

Vienna Fingers, barbeque chips, and ice cream, I thought of items that both of my sons could enjoy in their place.

As an example, my youngest son loves cereal (e.g., *Fruity Pebbles, Lucky Charms, Cinnamon Toast Crunch*, etc.) with 1 percent milk so I buy it for him to snack on. He also likes low-fat yogurt snacks, 1 percent milk with *Nestle Quick* chocolate added to it, and most fruits (e.g., bananas, grapes, applesauce, strawberries, etc.), so I try to keep these items on hand. My oldest son is a different story. He doesn't like milk, but he does like string cheese, and he will eat the cereals my youngest son likes *minus the milk of course*. Also, although he is not big on fruit, he will eat clementines and fruit cups of pears *if I make him*. They both like ginger snaps, *Chex Mix* (hot and spicy for my oldest and traditional for my youngest), *Goldfish, Teddy Grahams, Cheese-Its, Gripz, Social Tea Biscuits*, low-fat turkey pepperoni, *Ritz Crackers* (the whole-wheat ones), *Keebler Town Crackers*, etc. I try to pick things they both like, but foods that they are not as likely to lose their minds over and eat like they don't have any sense. *I want them to eat when they are hungry, and stop eating when they are not*. My husband will eat what's there, so I don't worry as much about him. This is a good thing because just trying to pick items that the boys like that won't cause me to overeat is enough of a challenge.

Whew! Heaven help the person who is trying to lose/maintain weight **and** has to buy and cook the food for the family as well! In most cases, it is the mom who is trying to juggle eating healthy with keeping hungry, growing, and busy people happy. It is hard to make sure everyone is well-fed, but not overeating or complaining/whining. Believe me, I hear a lot of mouth from people who want to tell me what to buy or cook. To be fair, I do occasionally ask my boys what snacks they would like me to buy after hearing them complain that I buy "lame" snacks. Then based on their *lame* responses, I will try to mix it up. *Oreos*, sodas, and ice cream are the most popular requests, but aside from holidays, special occasions (e.g., birthdays, good report cards, if my husband and I go out of town, if they have friends over, etc.) and vacations, I don't keep these items in the house. Of course they can indulge when they are at parties, social gatherings, or other people's houses—*just not at home on a regular basis*.

Before you think I am heartless, let me tell you, I have tried to keep the golden *Oreos* in the house, but each time the kids go to school, I eat over half of them! It's almost as if they call my name from the highest shelf in the house where I hide them from myself, and they taste *soooooo* good as I drink ice water from my mug. *Oh my goodness, I can just taste them now!* Then when my oldest son comes home, he asks, *"Is this all that's left?"* Each time I am so embarrassed, but I still laugh as I say, *"I told you I cannot be trusted with those things—It is all your fault!"* Also, I tried to keep barbeque chips (i.e., *Utz* or *Lay's Kettle Cooked Chips*) in the house because my husband likes them with sandwiches, but my youngest son and I kill the bags so fast that it just can't work. So no more! As a result, I walk a fine line between depriving people for my sake and making sure they have foods they like on a regular basis. However, for the most part, I have created an environment that is geared up for my success at maintaining a healthy weight as well as for teaching the kids how to eat like they have some sense.

Remember, *eating like you have some sense does not necessarily mean depriving yourself, it just means making the wisest, healthiest choice(s) you can at the time*. Sometimes these choices may not even be perceptible… As an example, when my boys eat toast, sandwiches, or homemade French toast, they are eating the *Healthy Life* low-calorie, whole-wheat bread I eat, and they have no complaints. Their burgers and barbeque sandwiches are often on low-fat, whole-wheat buns, but do they notice? Of course not. Also, although the main drink at our house is water, box drinks and Gatorades are still available when the boys play basketball or want them as snacks. So I do not feel guilty, especially when people still get *occasional* trips to *Dairy Queen, McDonald's,* and *Cold Stone Creamery, and* I know they eat junk at school. So trust me, no one is really being deprived. I am just balancing what we need versus what we want, and when this balancing act is done right, the quest to lose and maintain our weight becomes that much simpler. So it's basically all about the choices, my dear friend. *It's all about the choices…*

Behavior Modification Is Key

Are you starting to get the picture, or is the eating-like-you-have-some-sense concept still a little nebulous or hard to grasp? Just in case it is, a few more tips or examples on making better choices or changing your behavior

may be in order. What does it *really* mean to eat like you have some sense????
Yeah, yeah, I know I said it is about eating what you like in moderation,
making good choices and not depriving yourself, but how do you *really*
apply this to *your* life? What does it really entail? What do you really have
to do? Well, most of the effort lies in behavior modification—*creating new
and improved habits/patterns*. However, before you can successfully modify
your behavior, you must spend some time analyzing the existing eating
habits/patterns that make up your everyday life. Once you really *see* what
you are doing on a regular basis to sabotage your efforts to lose weight and
keep it off, you will be better able to change habits/patterns and ultimately
your behavior. *Only you can make the changes though.* To help facilitate your
efforts, I have put together yet another list of commonsense tips/ideas that
may help you get started with the task of modifying your behavior:

- Just because you are at an all-you-can-eat restaurant, *it does not literally*
  mean *you have to eat all you can.* You can still indulge in a *few* of the
  items that you most enjoy, but it should not be a free-for-all where you
  eat any and everything just because it is there or because you feel like
  you paid for it. Also, you don't *have to* clean your plate. After you have
  eaten a *reasonable amount* of the foods that you *really* love (they should fit
  on one plate—no more than one layer), ask yourself if you are full, and
  if you are, *STOP EATING!* Not saying you can't have seconds if you are
  still hungry, but if you are not (*really think about it*), don't eat anymore.
  Leave if you must, but **stop eating!** If you can't leave, just have some
  water or a cup of coffee while you wait.
- Just because someone else is eating does not mean you have to eat too!
  Even if the person offers you food repeatedly or tries to make you feel
  guilty—*you know whether you are hungry or not*, and you know whether
  or not you should be eating at that point. Believe me, it is OK just to
  sit and talk to someone while he or she eats or just sip on water/coffee
  while the person finishes, *especially if you have already eaten*. If you are not
  hungry, **DO NOT EAT!**
- Just because you are at the mall, it does not mean that you *have to* get
  a cookie, a cinnamon bun, pretzels, ice cream, or a smoothie. Having
  these high-calorie, high-fat indulgences are fine—maybe every fifth visit

to the mall, but *not every time.* This is something I tell my kids, who beg for *Cold Stone Creamery* every time we go to the mall, even offering to use their own money. As I tell them, you don't want this type of eating to become a habit or for it to be associated with even the most routine mall trip. When we do indulge in the *occasional* treat at these places, you can bet we will not have eaten a huge lunch or dinner and snacks beforehand! Get the picture? *These are rare treats.*

- Just because you are at the movies, *it does not mean you have to* get a huge soda, pretzel, candy, nachos, and/or popcorn *every* time. Sometimes one or more of these items can be OK, but not *every* time you go to the movies. In fact, you should try to eat before you get there because there is just too much to tempt you at the concession stands. Not only is it mostly high-fat, high-calorie and high-sodium junk (yeah, I said it), it is also ridiculously expensive! So now, I just split a bag of popcorn and a bottle of water with my husband or the kids. Before, a big bag of *M&Ms* and a soda was included with the popcorn, but not anymore. Can you relate? If so, make changes as needed.

- Just because you like a food/drink does not mean that it is in your best interest to eat it on a regular basis. In fact, there are some foods/drinks that should be relegated to the special occasion or vacation category. One example for us is *Edy's Cookies & Cream* ice cream. We can't have it in our house on a regular basis because we will eat it *every* day just because it is there and because it is so unbelievably good. I finally had to make the decision that I will only buy it on vacation, special occasions, or when the boys have their braces tightened and their teeth hurt. I have been told that I make the best milkshakes in the world using this ice cream, and I must agree. Be that as it may, even though I use 1 percent milk, these milkshakes are obviously treats that must stay in the special occasion category. *I don't care if the grocery store has a buy-one-get-one-free special going on!*

Another exception I also make on vacations is eating *McDonald's* sausage and egg *McGriddles* (I used to eat two, but I soon realized I never *need* two) and *Snickers* bars. I also enjoy *Starbucks* iced lemon pound cake and a café latte with sugar galore on special occasions. Although I love these treats, they must stay in the vacation or special occasion category for the most part. I cannot bring that type of eating home with me. Just like with Vegas, *what's done on vacation, stays on vacation.* This means that the eating habits from vacations, special occasions, or holidays should not become your normal routine. **You must get back to your normal eating habits as soon as possible.**

To further illustrate that point, I remember telling a fellow Southerner about the wonderful dinner I made one weekend: collard greens seasoned with bacon, vinegar, and jalapenos; corn bread; candied sweet potatoes; macaroni and cheese, and ribs. I was whining about how tired I was afterward because I only cook like that about four times a year, but the food was so good! As he was salivating, he said that cooking like that should be required every Sunday. I laughed and said that it is required eating every week only if you are trying to get hypertension, heart disease, and wind up overweight! We laughed, and he asked if I made my red velvet cake to go with it. I told him that I only make that for birthdays and holidays. It is such a rich cake that we cannot just sit around eating that wonderfully, fattening cake on a regular basis. Some items are really just for special occasions. So you *can* eat like you have some sense and enjoy your favorite rich and fatty foods, but you just can't do it on a regular basis. Do you have any foods that need to be put in the special occasion category? *I am sure you do.* If so, what are they, and what can you do to limit your contact with these foods on a regular basis? Think about it, and *make the necessary changes.*

* Just because a food or drink has a purpose, it does not give us permission to eat or drink it like it is going out of style. Sure nuts (e.g., walnuts, Brazil nuts, almonds, etc.) have the omega fatty acids we need to keep our hearts healthy, but because of their fat and calorie content, eating more than a handful a day could lead to trouble. Also, milk helps build strong bones, but can we just sit around drinking it all day without gaining weight? *I don't think so.* Sure juice is healthy and has added calcium these days, but it should still be in the occasional drink category as well. No matter what a food/drink's benefit is, you still have to keep in mind the fat/sugar/calories it contains. While I may have milk, juice, and

nuts under control, I did run into trouble with *Red Bull* about a year ago...

Because I struggle to stay awake after 9:30 most nights I am usually losing steam about the time my boys are getting ready for bed—*the time when I am finally free to do what I want to do (e.g., write, work on Web sites, surf the Web, etc.)*. During the day I am usually working jobs that pay the bills, and the rest of my "quality" awake time is devoted to kids' activities, homework, dinner, housework, exercise, spouse, etc. The nighttime seemed to be the right time to finally do what I wanted to do, if only I could stay awake... But I couldn't... I was very frustrated to say the least.

For most people coffee/sodas might be the answer, but I have some sort of resistance to caffeine. If I am sleepy, nothing can usually keep me awake. My family jokes that I have a sleep disorder. In fact, my husband has often said that if Oprah said she was coming to the house at midnight to bring me a billion dollars, I would probably sleep through it even if I had unlimited coffee/soda and even if he tried to wake me up! I hate to admit it, but he is right. Even in college during exams if I drank a pot of black coffee, I would still fall asleep—my stomach would be upset, but I would still be asleep. So when my cousin first told me about *Red Bull*, I thought it was the miracle solution to help me stay awake. At first it was because I could stay awake until 3:00 a.m. on one eight-ounce can. Of course I would be very tired the next day, but at least I was finally making progress!

This drink was also appealing because, as a person who does not drink alcohol, having a cold, sparkling drink in a champagne glass after the kids are in bed was a very nice treat. So the next thing you know, I was drinking as many as two eight-ounce cans a night! After about a month of this, instead of staying awake, I started to fall asleep before I could even finish one! Even when I could finish the second one, I would fall asleep immediately afterward! *What on earth had happened?* I have no idea why *Red Bull* stopped working for me, but I soon noticed the effect it had on my waistline in a *Cache* fitting room where I couldn't even zip up a size 6 dress that I wanted to buy. **Cache is my store,** and all of the clothes I buy there are a size 6—*nothing larger*. I took the dress off and left the store immediately. **Note:** *Don't get caught up in my size in this example, just focus on **your** goal size (whatever it may be), and adopt a **fight-to-stay-where-you-want-to-be** mentality. That's the purpose of this example…*

That did it! Not only was the *Red Bull not* keeping me awake, but I had gained weight from drinking so much (*it does contain quite a bit of sugar*). So my new habit had to go! Obviously my body needed the extra sleep. So I would just have to be more productive during the day (e.g., get people to help me more in the house, be more selective about what I do with my free time, etc.). So I *decided* to only have one 16.9-ounce *Red Bull* a week. It is my Friday night indulgence, but I cannot have it unless I walk to the store to get it. I still use a champagne glass, which makes it a special treat, but once it is gone, that is it until next week. Guess how I was rewarded for this behavior modification? The extra weight came off, and I was able to buy that dress from Cache *in a size 6* a few months later! Believe me, *when your habits change, your body will change too.* So, is there any habit you need to kick or drastically reduce your intake of? If so, *do it now!*

- Have you ever found yourself standing in front of a vending machine just to see what it has? I know I have! When we engage in this type of *window-shopping*, it usually means we are not hungry. Sometimes we are just bored and are looking to see if anything catches our fancy. I know I used to go to the vending machine at work around 2:30 every day. It gave me something to look forward to because I was bored, and having a soda and/or bag of popcorn seemed to help the afternoon go by quicker. *These are not good reasons to eat.* Just because a vending machine is accessible does not mean that you have to eat from it on a regular basis. So if you are doing this, just keep it moving, and go find some fruit if you are craving something sweet or a handful of nuts or a pickle if you are craving something salty (some pickles now have jalapeno or garlic flavoring, which I actually love). *Vending machines are not our friend.* An occasional treat is fine, but other than that, we must cut them loose. Make a clean break. *Do it now!*

I hope in all of the examples/tips I have given so far, you find a recurring theme: **Everything in moderation is the key to your success.** I don't know if you have noticed or not, but I am going out of my way *not* to tell you what you can't eat or have. This is because I want you to enjoy *what you like* in moderation. I don't want you to have a dieter's mentality—*one of deprivation or restriction.* Behavior modification can work for the long-term, but telling yourself you can never have something is not as likely to work for the long-term. Believe me, I know. I didn't eat chocolate for two years, and when I finally had it again (*see Wake-Up Call #3 in Chapter 3*), I literally lost my mind, and my weight soon reflected it.

So if I want chocolate, *I have chocolate.* However, to keep myself in check, I do set boundaries where chocolate items are concerned—no *Oreos, Chips Ahoy, Toll House* cookie dough, or candy bars in the house except for special occasions (*Halloween candy is an indulgence I allow until the end of November—then I give it away*). Another special occasion treat I still love dearly is *Keebler Fudge Covered Graham Crackers*, but I can only be trusted to eat them one week out of a month (as my grandmother used to say, "*You can catch on, can't you?*"). By the last day of that *special* week, all of the cookies are gone, and I have disciplined myself not to buy more until the next month. *Get the picture?* Eat what you want, just control *when, where,* and *how.* Talk to yourself, reason with yourself and make agreements as necessary. I may be crazy, but I do this quite a bit, and IT WORKS! Try it for yourself. What have you got to lose other than weight?

Eating Like You Have Some Sense

~ . ~ . ~ ~ . ~ . ~ . ~

In the last chapter I gave many ideas, examples, and suggestions on how and where you can make better choices in your eating and drinking. Better choices (*all won't be good, but they should definitely be better than what you are doing now*) are the cornerstone of the whole *eating-like-you-have-some-sense* concept. If you make *better* choices where your eating and drinking are concerned, losing and maintaining weight for the long-term will be that much easier. As I said before, eat *what* you want, just control **when, where,** and **how**. Basically all I am saying is to e*njoy the foods and drinks you like,* **in moderation.** What a novel idea! Like you haven't heard that one before! I know you have, and as you also already may know, this is often easier said than done. That's why the goal of this chapter is to arm you with the support and strategies you need to do this and to help you *really* get your eating under control once and for all. So without further delay, here are the strategies you need to really *eat like you have some sense:*

Eating-Like-You-Have-Some-Sense Strategy #1

To lose/maintain weight, you don't have to be perfect, but you do have to **be consistent where your eating/drinking habits are concerned.** The one thing that I know for sure is that the closer you can be to a creature of habit with your eating and drinking, the easier it will be for you to lose the weight and keep it off once and for all. The best way to do this is to eat three meals a day, around the same time every day. So you should *always* eat breakfast, lunch, *and* dinner, *especially breakfast* (even if you just eat yogurt or fruit). If you are a meal

159

skipper, **stop it**! *No meal skipping allowed!* I don't care whether you *think* you are hungry or not!

Contrary to what many dieters think, skipping meals does not save calories or get you closer to your weight loss goal. All it does is set you up to eat more food later, with a desperate sense of hunger that makes you feel justified to overeat. I know you have heard people justify eating huge meals by saying, *"This is the first meal I have had all day!"* Then you watch them eat the equivalent of two or more meals in one sitting. This type of behavior wreaks havoc on your metabolism. Going hungry all day and then eating huge meals at night makes your metabolism sluggish. Think of your metabolism as a fire, and imagine throwing a bunch of big logs into that fire all at once. That is obviously not the most efficient way to get/keep the fire going, and doing this consistently will cause your metabolism to burn slower than that of a person who eats reasonable-sized meals throughout the day. You could say that eating regularly keeps the metabolism "stoked" so calories are burned optimally throughout the day.

I believe this is why some people who struggle with their weight are frustrated when they compare their eating habits to those of a slimmer person who is consistently eating throughout the day (*three meals with a snack or two in between*). They often wonder why the slimmer person is seemingly able to eat more than they can and still maintain his or her weight. The conclusion often becomes that the slimmer person was just blessed with a faster metabolism. Well, I know there are a few people who may have been blessed with exceptionally fast metabolisms, but **most are not.** One of the secrets of slimmer people is the fact that they usually eat more consistently, which keeps the fire in their engines (*the metabolism*) stoked and burning optimally. Would you believe that sometimes, the more often you eat, the faster your metabolism is? It is true, and if you are going to lose weight and keep it off once and for all, you will definitely need your metabolism working as fast/optimally as it can.

OK, so how do you do that? Well the first thing you should do is come up with a list of foods that you enjoy that are healthy or at least relatively healthy that you can rotate for breakfast, lunch, and dinner on a daily/weekly/monthly basis. Then you need to make sure your day has enough structure to allow time for those meals—it may require a little planning, but it is well worth it. To get you started on both fronts, here are a few tips for each meal:

• **Breakfast**—I agree with whoever said that breakfast is the most important meal of the day. It is the meal that gets you and your metabolism going, and your goal should be to get your metabolism working like a well-oiled machine. *Fast-food/convenience store breakfast foods do not count*—they should definitely be in the once-in-a-while category, not for your everyday, *eat-like-you-have-some-sense* breakfast. Some of the choices for a healthy breakfast include: cereal (preferably whole-wheat and/or high-fiber) with low-fat milk; oatmeal with low-fat milk; scrambled eggs or omelets with cheese, vegetables, etc. cooked using a nonstick spray and with toast; yogurt and fruit; French toast (a couple of slices of whole-wheat bread dipped in an egg and cinnamon mix and fried using a nonstick spray); or cheese toast with jelly (use whole-wheat bread, toast it, and melt some shredded cheddar cheese on it in the oven or microwave), etc.

Of course this list is not exhaustive. There are other choices that could be just as healthy, if not healthier. I just wanted to give you a few examples to get you started. Did you notice that I didn't mention foods that require cream cheese or other items that are very high in fat/calories to taste good (e.g., bagels, grits, cream of wheat, etc.)? I am putting these in the occasional column because the potential for bad could outweigh the good/nutritional value. As an example, I love grits, but I only want them with eggs, bacon, and sausage, so I eat them maybe once or twice a month at the most, but **never** daily or weekly. So there are items that you can eat every day, while others should only be eaten every so often. Once you think of the healthy items you like, create a ritual that allows you to eat them consistently.

I have a morning ritual that I have been following for years to make sure I get breakfast during the week. As soon as I wake up, I put the 1 percent milk container in the freezer so that by the time I shower and put my contacts in, the milk is ice cold. I then put cereal (*my favorite mix is Honey Nut Cheerios, Raisin Bran, Frosted Mini-Wheats/Maple Sugar, and a sprinkling of Eggo Waffle/Maple Syrup cereal*) in a plastic cup (sixteen ounces or smaller), and I eat it in the bathroom while I do my hair and makeup. **Note:** *I don't care that the cereals I like have added sugar—they taste good, provide some nutritional benefit/fiber, keep me away from fast-food, and I feel really good and full for hours after eating them. That's all that matters to me.* By the time I am finished eating, my hair and makeup are done, and I am dressed. Before I walk out of the house, I drink a few shots of juice (e.g., prune, grapefruit, orange and/or acai) with my supplements (e.g., *One-A-Day Women's Formula*, a B-complex vitamin, vitamin E, flaxseed oil, fish oil, etc.).

I do this at least five days a week, and I am good until about 11:00 a.m. (*i.e., fully able to resist doughnuts, pastries, cake, and candy even if they are free or someone keeps offering!*). Then I grab a piece of fruit (usually a banana, but it could also be an orange, strawberries or grapes) and/or a cup of hot green tea (*with sugar of course*) or a couple of shots of juice (*e.g., carrot, pomegranate, etc.*), which holds me until lunch and keeps me from being so starved at lunch that I am tempted to overeat. This type of healthy snacking when *we are hungry*, helps keep our blood sugar stabilized and our metabolism stoked (burning efficiently). So eating when you are hungry is a good thing, but making the wisest choices as to what you actually eat will make all of the difference.

I am not saying there are not some days where I might allow myself to indulge in doughnuts, *McGriddles*, waffles, croissants or grits/eggs/bacon/sausage because I do enjoy them, but this **cannot** be more than a once or twice a week indulgence if I am trying to lose/maintain my weight. *Same goes for you.* So with that said, what healthy/relatively healthy items are you going to start eating for breakfast and as a late-morning snack on a regular basis?

_____

_____

_____

_____

_____

Give this a lot of thought because being consistently healthy with breakfast can be one of the greatest weapons in your weight loss/maintenance arsenal.

• **Lunch**—Even though breakfast is the most important meal of the day, I think lunch is very important in its own right because it sets the course for your whole afternoon. I say this because if you don't eat a good lunch, or you don't get lunch at all, you won't have the energy you need to finish the day strong. Your energy level will start to wane in the late afternoon— just when you may need it the most (e.g., as you are wrapping up your work, picking up/dropping off kids, looking at homework, making dinner, etc.). The afternoon is a time when we are often tempted to drink sodas or fatty concoctions from *Starbucks* or *Dunkin' Donuts*, eat snacks from vending machines or other high-fat, high-calorie junk that we should not be eating. However, eating a well-balanced lunch around the same time every day can help keep our blood sugar on an even keel so we can make it through that last busy stretch before dinner without eating something that we will regret.

When I worked in corporate environments lunchtime was often a troubling time as I wondered each day, *"What am I going to eat for lunch?"* Eating sandwiches, pizzas or other items from delis or fast-food restaurants grows old very fast. However, for millions of people this is a time when we spend a lot of money on overpriced, fatty, greasy, high-calorie, high-sodium, unhealthy foolishness that takes us further and further away from our weight loss goals. I think this happens because we are hungry, pressed for time, and cannot think of anything better to eat. If you are one of those people popping a frozen entrée into the microwave, don't think you are off the hook because your food may very well fall into the unhealthy foolishness category as well. I say this because many of those entrees are filled with sodium to preserve them as well as to make them taste like you are eating something real. Also, they may not be as filling or nutritious as a freshly prepared meal. *So what's a hungry person trying to eat like they have some sense supposed to do?*

YOU HAVE TO PLAN! You have to take matters into your own hands and be prepared before lunch with an idea of what you are going to eat. You cannot afford to wait until you are hungry, stressed and pressed for time. Because everyone is different, there are a number of ways to prepare for this lunchtime crisis. The people who enjoy eating leftovers from last night's dinner, which is perfectly fine, obviously have an advantage as long as the meals do not include a large amount of fried/fatty foods or serving sizes that cause you to eat beyond the point of being full. Also, they must include some fruits and vegetables. If you are that *left-over-lunch-loving* person, get out the Tupperware, and take it with you! This will save you time, money, and aggravation, and you can eat whenever you are ready.

Unfortunately this is not me—I don't want to eat what I had for dinner last night for lunch. *I just don't.* Am I the only one? In case I am not, people like us will need to be especially prepared. We have to identify healthy/reasonably healthy items we like to eat for lunch, and make sure we have the necessary items available when we are hungry. If you are very disciplined (*I am not*), you could make food the night before (e.g., grilled or baked chicken/fish, rice, pasta, or regular salads, etc.), and pack it up so it is ready for the next day. If that is you, great! Just be sure to pack all of the necessary condiments (e.g., dressing, sauces, etc.) to go with it (*use them sparingly—just enough to taste*). *You must be prepared so you don't have any excuse to eat something other than what you brought.*

I just am not disciplined enough to make preparations the night before like this, and I don't like to eat dinner-type foods during the day, so I am left preparing simple meals that kids generally eat… Even though I am in my forties, *I LOVE TO EAT PEANUT BUTTER AND JELLY SANDWICHES* at least two to three times a week! Sometimes more. In fact, when I worked in corporate environments, I would take a loaf of whole-wheat, low-fat bread (preferably *Healthy Life*, but *Wonder Lite* will do), a jar of *Skippy* or *Peter Pan* chunky peanut butter and a squeeze bottle of *Welch's* grape jelly to make lunches during the week. Only these brands will do, and *the jelly has to be cold.* When everything is right, it is one of my favorite lunches. I kid you not! I think I am a big kid because eating that sandwich while drinking ice cold water from my mug has me closing my eyes and licking the jelly from my fingers! Mesquite or barbeque chips with ridges are the best tasting combination with it, but I had to put the chips away because I can't eat just one serving. Instead I grab at least two fruits (e.g., a banana, orange, clementine, peach, grapes, strawberries, etc.) and a pickle spear (garlic flavored) or a container of *Campbell's* vegetable, alphabet soup. Having these items handy at all times ensures that I never have to think about what I am going to eat, which keeps me from eating out more than once or twice a week. Also, when other people are going to *McDonald's, Taco Bell, Popeyes* or *KFC*, I am not tempted. Because I know what I like, and I make sure I keep it handy.

This will be your secret as well—*figure out what you like, and keep it on hand* so you can eat a lunch you prepare at least three or four times a week, if not more. I know everyone does not like peanut butter and jelly, but what about a BLT (bacon, lettuce, and tomato sandwich); a sandwich/sub with lean deli meats, veggies, mustard, and seasonings; grilled cheese and/ or low-sodium, vegetable-based canned soups? Try mixing and matching these items, and add fruits, vegetables, or salads to make it a well-balanced meal. For those of you who may be wondering, you can add a bag of chips to the mix, but it should be the single serving bags (sometimes you see them sold for twenty-five cents or in bulk containers in grocery stores), not the huge bags sold in delis/convenience stores. If you get those, try to save half for another day or share it with someone. Also, try drinking water with your lunch or cutting the sweetened drinks down to half your normal size. Your success lies in your choices, but if you choose relatively healthy items that you like and always have them available, you should be in good shape, *literally*. So now all you have to do is come up with healthy/relatively healthy items that you enjoy eating for lunch:

_____

_____

_____

_____

_____

I think I have given you enough information to get the ball rolling, but let's face it, eating what you prepare will get boring if you do it every day. Another one of the keys to your long-term success is making sure you are enjoying what you eat for lunch, so eating out for lunch is still allowed (*occasionally* anyway). As a result, you should prepare for this as well with a few guidelines to help you make good choices as you visit restaurants for lunch:

o   Try to limit your eating out to no more than once or twice a week for the most part. Some weeks you may go out three times, but try not to do it consistently.

o   Also, as you are going out, fast-food restaurants and convenience stores would not be my first choice for you. However, if you find yourself at a fast-food restaurant be very conservative: get the smallest burger they have, no extra cheese, no extra meat, don't add chili; get the smallest order of nuggets/tenders/strips they have; get the small fries or just skip them altogether, and eat fruit with your meal; *don't super-size ANYTHING*; don't get the combo (drink water if you can); don't get anything two-for-one; don't add a shake; and don't get dessert. *Just stay focused on your goals, and get outta there!*

o   As with the lunches you prepare, avoid fatty sauces, dressings and condiments. Go very easy on these items, only use the minimum amount needed for taste. I read once that salad dressing accounts for a large percentage of the fat women consume. So keep your lunches as healthy as you can by not asking for extra dressing, cheese and/or meat for your salads. *If you can't do this, then maybe you should choose fruit instead of a salad.*

I have heard that we should eat breakfast like a king/queen, lunch like a prince/princess, and dinner like a pauper, but I am not sure if I fully agree because I don't think breakfast and lunch should be very heavy meals. If they are, a lot of us will be walking around feeling very sluggish. However, I do agree that we should not starve ourselves during the day, saving the heavy eating for the evening just when your activity is starting to wind down. Many people do this because they skip meals, which means they are extremely hungry by the time lunch or dinner rolls around. I know a lot of people skip breakfast because they are rushed to get out of the house in the morning, but you can either take breakfast with you, or find ways to squeeze it into your morning routine like I have. *Either way, you cannot afford to skip these two important meals.*

Now that you have breakfast, a late-morning snack, and lunch out of the way, it is time to prepare for the home stretch—*late afternoon and evening*, the time of the day where we run into the most trouble. This is the time when we are most likely to grab a candy bar or go to *Dunkin' Donuts* for some late afternoon snack. *Contrary to what we hear in commercials, there is no "new meal" between lunch and dinner!* Don't get me wrong, there is definitely room for snacks, especially healthy items, but no room *or* need to create a new meal! If you have heard/thought about this, please forget all about it! A better choice for afternoon snacks might be: fruit (e.g., orange, banana, raisins, prunes, etc.), cut-up veggies, nuts (e.g., walnuts, sunflower seeds, Brazil nuts, etc.), yogurt, a cup of green tea or 100 percent juice, etc. Try to squeeze in something healthy that will help you make it until dinner. I usually grab a handful of walnuts/sunflower seeds/macadamias/raisins mixed together with a shot of low-sodium V-8 juice. It is a nice mix of sweet and salty tastes, and I feel better than I would if I ate a candy bar.

- **Dinner**—This is the meal where we are most likely to get into trouble because after a long, stressful day, we are tired and hungry, *especially if we did not eat consistently throughout the day.* At this time of the day our thinking/creativity is at an all-time low, and some of the demands placed on our time are at an all-time high (e.g., deadlines, commuting, picking people up, dropping people off, cooking, doing housework, checking homework, etc.). This is also the time when we are most likely to justify eating more to make up for how good we were earlier or for how hectic the day was. *This is not the time to do that,* especially since your calorie burning potential for the evening is the lowest it probably is all day. Your activity/metabolism is winding down, and so should your heavy eating.

There are a lot of pitfalls that wait for us at dinner, but one of the best ways to safeguard against bad choices and overeating is to plan ahead. You do this by having a few relatively healthy recipes that you can rotate and keep the ingredients on hand. This will make you more likely to cook at home instead of eat out, which will save you calories, fat, and money! Here are some of the meals I rotate during the week:

o   Beef tacos/burritos/quesadillas (turkey or chicken breasts can also be used) topped with lettuce, tomatoes and cheese served with green beans

o   Barbeque sandwiches (made from chicken breasts or a pork roast seasoned with products from *Famous Dave's*) on whole-wheat buns, corn, and broccoli

o   Spaghetti casserole, garlic bread, a green vegetable or salad and carrots

o   Barbeque chicken (drumsticks or wings), rice, and a green and yellow vegetable

o   Fried tilapia and baked salmon, biscuits and a green and yellow vegetable

o   Cabbage, corn bread, Polska Kielbasa, chicken and/or fish, and baked sweet potatoes

o   Homemade, beef vegetable soup, corn bread and baked sweet potatoes

o   Lean, ground beef cheeseburgers on whole-wheat buns with Campbell's soup for the kids, and a green/yellow vegetable for us (*tater tots are OK occasionally*)

o   Turnips or greens, cornbread, barbeque ribs, and candied sweet potatoes

o   Low-country boil (a spicy gumbo type dish with shrimp, Polska Kielbasa, red potatoes and corn), rice, and a green vegetable

Hey, I never said I was a gourmet chef, but these are just a few of the meals I rotate that can last at least two or three days. Say if I cook on Sunday, *I don't want to cook again until Tuesday*, and after that, I don't want to cook until Saturday or Sunday! That is my normal pattern. Who has time or wants to cook every day? *I know I don't!* This is why I came up with a number of meals that I can make during the week that mix in foods we like and some things that we don't like as much. However, they are relatively healthy, and I usually buy the ingredients in advance. Having the ingredients on hand makes things so much easier because you don't have to run to the store each time you cook, and you can get started/finish faster. That is one of the secrets to successfully eating *healthier* dinners at home—*be prepared,* so the effort is not overwhelming.

I know if you don't really like to cook, coming up with a list of more than a few meals can be hard. *Especially when you are cooking for more than two people.* Unfortunately my list is based on trying to please four picky people (*well, really only three of us are picky*). It is hard to do, but *it can be done.* You can start by coming up with a list of entrees or main courses (e.g., a casserole, pasta, or meat) that you and your family enjoy:

_____

_____

_____

_____

_____

Once you have your list, build meals around it by adding at least two vegetables such as: broccoli and carrots, green beans and corn, etc. Vary the vegetables as often as you can, and add a vegetable-based soup whenever possible. You can also add bread or a starch as it makes sense. I know I told you that I am not a carb-conscious person who is reading labels and obsessing about what foods can be eaten together. However, I am a trade-off person, which means that I try to make wise decisions for me and my family as I prepare dinner. As a result, I try to avoid processed, pre-made foods such as hot dogs, canned items, and frozen dinners (*too much sodium, preservatives, and fat*), and I try to limit *most* dinners to only one starch. As an example, we only have bread with dinner a few times a week (e.g., corn bread, biscuits, rolls, etc.), and when we do, there is no butter anywhere to be found. Also, if we have bread at dinner, there is usually no rice, corn, or white potatoes. Having more than one of these items in a regular meal seems too heavy, and *it just feels like your body would waste no time converting those extra carbs/starches into fat.* Can I prove that this is what happens physiologically? Of course not, but if I were you, I would not be sitting around eating bread and rice or mashed potatoes in the same meal! Instead, I would replace the extra starch or bread with more vegetables whenever possible. *Aha!* More vegetables, less bread/starches, and drinking lots of water with your meal will put you closer to your goals.

Whew, explaining how to be consistent with your meals is a hard thing to do. *I have not even addressed strategies for eating at restaurants (I will do that later)!* Regardless, I think you have enough information to get started with the task of preparing and making selections for breakfast, lunch, mid-morning snacks, dinner and mid-afternoon snacks. Unfortunately, this is not all the eating we will do in a day… There is the matter of after-dinner/late-night snacking, which is often the downfall of the best-laid, healthy eating, weight loss plans. It is a tricky area that I will cover *fully* in a later strategy. However, for those of you that do not struggle in this area, feel free to grab a snack after dinner such as a single-serving frozen treat (i.e., *Dreamsicle*, *Fudgesicle*, sorbet, sherbet, etc.), a piece of chocolate or caramel, or some other limited-serving treat. *Then stop there.* Clean up the kitchen, brush your teeth—do whatever it takes to end the eating for the evening. If you need a glass/cup of milk, tea, juice or coffee, *have it.* Also, have all of the water you want, but the eating for the day is over. You enjoyed a day of good food that you enjoy, now it is time to do something else!

Note: You may want to invest in or choose smaller plates for lunch and dinner. Remember, *the larger the plate, the larger the portions—the smaller the plate, the smaller the portions.* Something as simple as using a smaller plate can actually trick you into eating less.

Eating-Like-You Have-Some-Sense Strategy #2

What if I told you that drinking a full glass of water before each meal could cause you to eat 25 percent less at each meal, enabling you to lose/keep off five extra pounds each year? *Would you do it?* Well I can't promise you these types of results because every person's body *and* metabolism are different. However, there is a good chance that it *could* happen. So instead of *gaining* a few pounds each year like the average person, *especially those over thirty*, you could gradually *lose* weight and possibly cause your metabolism to burn more efficiently, flush toxins from your body, and have clearer, younger looking skin. Why not take a chance? *What have you got to lose other than weight?*

So for all of these reasons, I say you should **drink water more than any other drink**. I think eight to ten glasses a day is our best bet. Sodas and alcohol are such a waste of calories (*yeah, I said it*), so consumption of these items should be kept to an absolute minimum. I see so many people out in restaurants and clubs drinking large sodas, frothy-looking drinks with whipped cream, huge daiquiris and all sorts of sweetened drinks. Think about it, twenty ounces of soda or a sweetened drink is too much, *especially for children*. If you have two or three of these drinks, you could consume more calories than you normally would in a meal. **These calories add up**, and if we are not careful, they could wind up helping us pack on unwanted pounds. So our safest, healthiest best is to drink water at least 90 percent of the time. The other 10 percent of the time you can still enjoy milk, juice, tea and your favorite drinks (*in that order*), but make your refills water. *I don't care if refills are free.* **Water is really one of your body's best friends.**

Once you get used to drinking water, you will find it to be such a refreshing drink. I am a self-confessed water-a-holic. As long as it is ice cold, I enjoy sipping it all day. It took me years to get to this point, but now I can't even function if I don't have a cup or mug of ice water close by. I cannot even stand the feeling of a dry mouth/thirst anymore because I am used to drinking so much water. This is a good thing because sometimes we can confuse thirst with hunger. *Can you believe that there are times where you think you are hungry, but you are really thirsty?* Water plays a major role in eating and acting like you have some sense. I know for a fact that it helps me eat less/get full faster, keeps me very regular, and it seems to help keep my skin relatively bump/zit-free. Also, I have never had a urinary tract infection even though I don't drink cranberry juice. *Water really is a miracle drink for you and your kids!*

For those of you who are still adamant about not liking to drink water—it truly is an acquired taste—but let me ask you this, did you like broccoli or other yucky vegetables you like today the first time you tried them? *Did you like alcohol the first few times you tried it?* In most cases, you did not. You started to like these things after trying them over a period of time. So the same goes for water—you just have to keep trying it. Add ice or orange/lemon slices to it, or drink it warm or cold. Whatever works for you, *it doesn't matter.* Do you like the taste of most medicines? Of course, not, but if they help you reach your goals, you will take them, right? Again, so it goes with water. **No ifs, ands, or buts about it, you gotta drink it!** Are you still fighting me on this? If so, give it a try when you are eating sweets or carbohydrates. This is how I got started and how I enjoy it best. I have to admit that I don't enjoy it as much when I am snacking on fruit (e.g., oranges, grapes, or apples) or right after drinking juice. I usually wait until after the taste of the fruit is gone. If this has been the case for you, give it another try.

Now that you are ready to try it, a good strategy to start with is to have water after breakfast as well as with lunch and dinner. A good rule is to drink at least *two sips for each bite you chew*. This slows your eating down, so you get full faster. As a result, you will eat less, and over time you *will* lose weight! So get you a big mug (*I bought a sixty-four-ounce insulated Coke mug with a straw from Wal-Mart*) or glass for work and for home, and get to sipping! The only downside I can think of for this water addiction is the fact that I go to the restroom a lot, but hopefully this means that my kidneys have major help flushing toxins out of my system.

One last important note: **Drinking water will not kill you or** *your kids*, and you are not a bad parent if water is the major drink you serve at home (*I am not talking about for infants/toddlers*). Many adults think that giving kids water is a form of a punishment. I assure you, *it is not*. In fact, it is a healthier choice in terms of their teeth and weight. Sure they can have *Kool-Aid* or soda *occasionally*, but these items should be considered as treats, *not the norm or something they feel entitled to*. One of the main reasons I bought a refrigerator with filtered ice and water was so the kids could easily grab water whenever they are thirsty. At that point I stopped making pitchers of *Kool-Aid every* week. Instead, I buy the single-serving packets of *Crystal Light* and box drinks for them to enjoy *occasionally*. I should feel guilty since I grew up drinking *Kool-Aid* almost every day of my life. However, I wound up with more cavities than I care to admit, a weight problem, and I never learned to really appreciate water. Now I believe water is one of our best friends, *especially as we lose and maintain our weight*.

Eating-Like-You-Have-Some-Sense Strategy #3

What if someone told you there was an anti-cancer pill that could reduce your chances of getting cancer—would you take it? Of course you would, but unfortunately there is no such pill. However, fruits, vegetables, nuts, and whole-grains are foods that have actually been shown to reduce the incidence of cancer and heart disease, but many of us still won't eat them on a regular basis. As I counsel (*nag*) my oldest son, who does not like fruit, I actually tell him that God gave us these foods as natural cancer and disease fighters. So, at some point, all of us are going to have to **make better, healthier food choices on a regular basis**. That point should be sooner rather than later, especially if you want to lose weight and live healthier. One of the other added benefits is the fact that *they help you feel fuller faster, so you will eat less.*

If all of these foods have such nutritional benefits, why is it that we tend to shy away from them? Well sometimes it has to do with taste or what we have become accustomed to eating. Other times, it may also have to do with a focus or preoccupation on calories. As an example, a woman might substitute a diet soda for a cup of orange juice or two cookies in place of a banana in order to avoid the calories these healthy items have. Although you may be saving calories, you are losing out on the nutritional benefit. I think this mind-set explains why some people trying to lose weight also give up foods such as: low-fat milk, yogurt, peanut butter, raisins, and heart-healthy nuts like almonds and walnuts. These items are forsaken because they have more calories than some of the processed snack items. You cannot compare the calories in a candy bar with those of a peanut butter and jelly sandwich on low-fat, whole-wheat bread. You are so much better off with the sandwich. Also, a doughnut may have the same calories as a bowl of cereal with low-fat milk, but it is no match for the fiber, calcium, vitamin D, **and** the fuller feeling that you will get from eating the cereal. *There really is no contest.*

So, better food choices are definitely in order. On a given day you may want to indulge, and that is OK, but over the long-term these are not substitutes you should make on a regular basis. An example of a better choice would be to have three slices of cheese toast on low-fat, whole-wheat bread instead of two *Pop-Tarts*. From a fiber and calcium perspective, the cheese toast is a clear winner, especially if you use low-fat cheese. *All calories are not equal, so our focus needs to be on nutrition, not calories.* I don't care if diet sodas are calorie-free, *they are no substitute for water, juice, or milk*—healthy drinks *or* flavored acid, *hmmm, let me think.*

I must admit I do understand how we wound up with this preoccupation with calories and why we are willing to trade nutrition to save calories. On the surface, it can seem like the fastest way to reach our weight loss goals. However, in the long-run it is not because, as I said before, *the way you eat to lose weight must be the way you are prepared to eat for a lifetime.* Also, this calorie-conscious philosophy can cause some of us to be scared to eat nuts, bananas, and dairy because of the calories/fat. However, these same people are often not scared to eat ice cream, chips, and fast-food. You won't believe how many people seem alarmed when I admit to eating peanut butter on a regular basis. *Do you know how many calories peanut butter has per tablespoon, they ask?* Not really, and to be honest, I *don't care* because I only use a layer thick enough where I can taste it on my sandwich. *I love it, and I will never give it up!* I also love walnuts, macadamias, and sunflower seeds, so I eat them *in moderation*, with a clear conscience. So I just laugh when people give me a hard time about it, but I also laugh as I realize that these same people won't think twice about eating a *Big Mac or Whopper* with fries and a large *Coke.* Isn't it funny that they will shy away from eating a handful of walnuts or almonds even though both contain healthy omega-3 fats and vitamin E, but they are not shy about eating fast food?

This needs to change... So let's get our priorities straight, and start eating based on nutrition and *not on calories.* Here are a few tips to help you with this:

- Add as much roughage and natural fiber to your daily meals as possible. I know some people may not like whole-wheat or grain products, but an occasional sandwich on whole-wheat, some whole-wheat/whole-grain cereal mixed in with your favorite cereal or brown rice will not kill you. In fact, it could help improve your overall health.
- *A day without fruits and vegetables is a no-no.* Think of fruits and vegetables as cancer fighters. They may not be a cure-all for cancer, but they give your body a fighting chance to protect itself. One of the ways that I can easily get three or four servings out of the way is by eating vegetable soup (homemade or *Campbell's*) with lunch or for dinner a few days a week. Otherwise, add at least two fruits/veggies or a salad to lunch and dinner. Also substitute fruits/veggies for snacks throughout the day. A few shots of 100 percent juice with meals or snacks, or as a late-night snack also helps. That is

eating pretty much what you want for breakfast, whatever sandwich you want for lunch, and whatever main course you like for dinner, you are just bringing the vegetables/fruits in on the side so you can get your daily helping of "cancer fighters."

- When incorporating vegetables into your diet, try to mix them up as much as you can... If you have broccoli, green beans and corn one week, the next week try to have salad, cabbage, and sweet potatoes. Maybe spinach, collard greens, or asparagus and carrots the next. Try to rotate the vegetables you like so you won't get bored and your diet is well-rounded. At least five nights a week, make sure you have at least one green vegetable (e.g., spinach, broccoli, greens, cabbage, green beans, etc.) and one yellow/red vegetable (e.g., corn, carrots, peppers, sweet potatoes, etc.). Fresh is best, but frozen works too—I don't want to be obsessive like some of the health advocates who frown on eating frozen vegetables. In a country that is moving away from eating more than a handful of vegetables in a week, I think it is best to just *start eating vegetables any way you can!*
- Also, don't forget to take a multi-vitamin supplement to address any dietary deficiencies.

Many ask why cancer is so prevalent in this country, and I really believe the answer lies in the fact that many of us are not being good stewards over the bodies we have been given. We are choosing foods and drinks based on calories or taste, not nutrition. This may help us to be slimmer, but definitely not healthier. Remember, *we are eating to live, not living to eat*, so our focus must be on living the healthiest life we can. Unfortunately, most people wait until they have a disease or condition before they start to eat and live healthier, but I am challenging you *and myself* to start now! We only get one life and one body, so let's make better choices today.

Eating-Like-You-Have-Some-Sense Strategy #4

Once you get full, stop eating and drinking. *Don't just keep eating until you clean your plate or until you are stuffed.* Of course, we know this is not as easy as it sounds. Regardless, you have to do it if you sincerely want to lose weight or maintain your current weight. Your stomach is a muscle, and when you regularly *eat beyond the point of being full*, it can stretch, which over time will require you to eat more to actually fill it up. So if you have been overeating for years, your stomach is probably larger than the average person's. As a result, you may need to begin efforts to shrink it back by learning to eat less, not drastic, *like on a diet* "less," but *eating like you have some sense* "less." Say if you normally eat all of the fries with a meal, try eating only half. Instead of having three pieces of chicken with dinner, try having one or two… If you would normally drink a twenty- or thirty-two-ounce soda with a meal, try to drink a twelve- or sixteen-ounce soda instead. If you are still thirsty, ask for water. Also, if you normally go back for thirds at dinner, try to stop at seconds or only a single helping…

These are just a few examples of how you can cut back while still enjoying your usual meals. I am sure you can think of other ways to cut back even more if you try. In the meantime, just try to use common sense when eating and deciding when you are full—*it should not take five pieces of chicken to fill you up!* If it does, your meal needs to be more balanced (e.g., more vegetables, soup, water, etc.), or you are eating out of taste or for some other reason. We must get to the point where we know our bodies well enough to know when we are full. Then we won't need to waste time weighing or measuring food. There are millions of people around the world, who are at a healthy weight, who have never weighed their food or cared to look at the caloric content on the back of a package. *This information is irrelevant when your eating is under control.*

It is also important to note that the older we get, the less we should be eating. I have heard that people who live longer tend to eat less as they age—*not more.* This is a good thing for all of the systems of your body, and as you eat less, your stomach starts to shrink. I have found this to be the case for me over the years as well. Here are few examples:

- I used to eat all the meat in an order of General Tso's chicken with three egg rolls, but now I am full after eating about a fourth or a half of the meat with no egg rolls.
- It used to be nothing for me to eat three drumsticks at dinner, but now I can only eat one or two without feeling stuffed.
- I used to be able to eat a whole individual pizza (e.g., Bertucci's or California Pizza Kitchen, etc.), but now I can barely eat half, and the rest comes home for the next day.

- At one point, I could eat a full bacon cheeseburger and fries from Champps or Sweetwater's, but now I have to take half home. Many times I don't even order fries.

Even though I drink a lot of water with my meals, I am still amazed at how my ability to eat has changed. My sons laugh and make jokes about how quickly I get full. They say my stomach is the size of a bird's. Well, let's not get crazy, but I have noticed that the less I overeat, the less food it takes for me to get full. *Jackpot!* That is what we want—*to be able to eat the foods we enjoy without overeating* **and** *without feeling deprived.* This means fewer calories and less fat, with the same enjoyment. However, the surprising long-term reward is weight loss/maintenance. So although there is no dieting, fewer calories are being consumed while the same types of foods are being eaten and the same restaurants are being visited... However, now we are getting closer to our goal of eating and acting like we have some sense.

Eating-Like-You-Have-Some-Sense Strategy #5
The more meals you can prepare/eat at home the better. A little planning is definitely required to help you do this consistently. Try to plan meals in advance whenever possible. Then take a trip to the grocery store to stock up on foods that you can eat for breakfast, lunch, and dinner, as well as snacks to keep *at home and at work* (e.g., cereal, oatmeal, bread, fruit, vegetables, juice, lean meats, yogurt, etc.). As you do this, try to avoid frozen/prepared meals. I know sometimes they can be convenient, especially for lunch and dinner, but you should not be eating them more than once or twice a week. These meals are often high in sodium and fat, and they are often not as filling as foods that you would prepare at home yourself. In my opinion, they are not *real* food, so they may not leave you as satisfied. Not only that, but many of these items do not provide a balanced meal. I am sure some of them are fine and healthy, but they would not be my first choice for you if you asked my opinion.

Regardless of the foods you buy, the whole process of deciding what to eat is so much easier when you have food already on hand. A meal where this preparation really pays off is dinner, especially if you make meals that last for at least two nights. This way you are not always wondering what to make/have for dinner, and you are more likely to eat less *and* healthier. Even if you have to take a cooking class (*I probably should*) or get tips from friends/family, you should cook your own food as often as possible. As an example, a piece of barbeque chicken, a serving of green beans, an ear of corn, and a roll for dinner would probably be more satisfying and possibly healthier than the average restaurant or frozen food dinner. You will notice that I tend to keep meals simple. One of the reasons is because I am not a very skilled cook, but I also believe keeping things simple makes it easier to eat like you have some sense. I know you have to do what works for you, but the simpler you keep things, the better.

Speaking of keeping things simple… When I am kicking off a lighter eating campaign, usually after pigging out on vacations or over holidays such as Christmas/Thanksgiving or before trips/vacations, I usually make a big pot of vegetable soup (*my mother-in-law's recipe*). Then for about three nights, I eat a big bowl of it with lots of hot sauce/pepper and a piece of cornbread crumbled in it, as well as a plain baked sweet potato. *This is so good!* Any vegetable-based soup will work just as well, but I can share the recipe for anyone who is interested on www.CarolynGrayInternational.com. This is such a good way to get things started off right *and* to keep you from worrying about what you are going to eat for dinner for at least a few nights.

Eating-Like-You-Have-Some-Sense Strategy #6

The reason I think my weight loss/maintenance plan has worked for me over the years is because it allows me to basically eat what I want—*foods that I already like and really enjoy. You can't really succeed on any plan, for the long-term, if you can't enjoy the foods you like.* With that said, I think you should make it a point to *only eat foods that you really, really like.* **Never eat just to eat.** My motto is "Eat What You Like," and if you don't *really, really* like something, **Don't Eat It!** Over the years I have seen people eating foods that don't look very appetizing, and I have often asked, "*How is it?*" Do you know how they usually respond? They usually make a face and say, "*Ah, it's just OK.*" So I ask, "*Then why are you eating it?*" My thing is why waste calories on something that you are not *really, really* enjoying?

As soon as I realize a food/meal is "just OK," I stop eating and try to find something that I truly want to eat, even if it means I have to wait until I get home.

Although I don't believe in counting calories, I also do not believe in *wasting* calories on something that I don't have a burning desire to eat. This philosophy is extremely helpful when you go to social events or get-togethers where there are large amounts of foods available. In many cases you may only really like or want to eat a few items, but the fear of hurting someone's feelings or being singled out for not eating like everyone else can cause you to eat *out of guilt*. **No matter who it is, I say don't do it.** Believe me, I have been in this situation many times before, and after years of feeling guilty and uncomfortable, I have decided just to say no or discretely eat only the things I like and keep it moving. I must admit it did take me a while to get to this point…

As an example, every Thanksgiving we have dinner at my mother-in-law's house. In the early days of my marriage I used to feel guilty when people asked me why I didn't have more food on my plate. I didn't want to hurt their feelings, so I wouldn't admit that I didn't like certain foods. Sometimes I would nibble a little and pretend to eat, but when they weren't looking, my husband and I would switch plates, or I would discretely throw it away. After a while, I asked myself, "Why am I being dishonest and wasteful?" I finally just started saying, "*No thank you.*" If people asked why, I would just say I was full. If they pressed further, I finally started honestly saying, *I don't like this or that (i.e., gravy, turkey, corn pudding, stuffing, macaroni, etc.).* These are obviously last resort answers, but you know how some people can get really pushy in their efforts to get you to eat what they are eating. This is my body, and it is *my* decision what I choose to put in it. **Case closed.** *The same should go for you as well!*

I think this is one of the reasons why I usually don't gain weight during Thanksgiving. Many of my sisters-in-law laugh when they see my plate—I have greens/green beans, bread, ham, and maybe sweet potatoes, and I drink water. Then I eat a few pieces of the red velvet cake that I bring (*my favorite*). That's it! I don't like cranberry sauce, casseroles, or a lot of store-bought cakes and pies, *so I choose not to eat these things.* I don't announce it—*no one needs to know my reasons/motivation.* Along with that, if something I put on my plate is not good or I don't like it, I discretely get rid of it. *Our bodies are not garbage disposals*, and it does not help starving people around the world for us to eat things that we don't like. I don't think we should be wasteful, but we have to be very selective about what we actually eat. There is just so much temptation to overeat that only eating foods we really like can help limit some of the overeating that we usually do. *This will ultimately lead to pounds lost or at least kept off.*

Eating-Like-You-Have-Some-Sense Strategy #7

In addition to strategy #6... **Just because food/drinks are free or available, you don't have to eat *or* drink them.** I don't care if cocoa, coffee (*only a problem if you use lots of sugar—this is one of my weaknesses*), or soda is in unlimited supply at work (*it used to be when I worked on a project at Freddie Mac*). If these indulgences are keeping you from reaching your weight loss goals, then *leave 'em alone.* It is doesn't matter if a restaurant has free refills on sodas or fries—*do you really need a refill of soda or sweetened drinks after you have already had one or two? Do you really need more fries? The answer is no.* Because we are offered so many foods and drinks that we really don't need, it might be worthwhile to practice saying *no.* This will help us to be ready to answer *firmly* and *quickly* when we are offered things that we are not really dying to have or we just plain old do not need...

As an example, I remember being in a drive-thru, and someone made a mistake with our order, so they offered me a free soda to make up for it. So I said, "*Thanks anyway, but may I have a cup of ice water instead?*" The person asked me if I was sure and looked at me like I was crazy, and so did my kids! *Who cares! If we don't need something, I don't care if it is free, we still don't need it.* No matter how good soda tastes or how manufacturers dress it up, you are drinking sweetened acid with *no* nutritional value!!!! *Who needs almost three hundred wasted calories?*

Another example of wasted calories could be if you walk into the kitchen at work, and someone has brought in a chocolate Halloween cake with orange whipped cream frosting that looks mildly interesting. **You do not have to eat it just because you see it.** Even if someone says, "*Have some,*" and *especially* if you have already eaten breakfast or just had a pastry that your boss brought in at a staff meeting. You know I am speaking from experience on this, right? I know so many people who may not necessarily have a burning desire to eat a piece of cake at 10:30 a.m., but they might *just because it is there*. There was a time when I would just eat a piece of cake because it was there, and I would think, "*Why not?*" Well there are good reasons why we shouldn't: 1) Because there may be other things we will want to eat later that we will probably enjoy more; or 2) Because we know that as we try to eat normally during the day, this treat will not help us reach our weight loss goals, basically it is what I call *a waste of calories*.

As you develop a habit of turning down these types of foods, *ones that are just there*, you will find your resolve getting stronger. Then it will be much easier to **only indulge in snacks that you have a burning desire to eat**. This means that you are still eating what you want, but *you are not eating any and everything that you see*, which will ultimately lead to weight loss or maintenance over the long-term. *This is what you want...* Because the whole decision-making process can be a tricky, I have created a model to help make it easier for you to decide whether *to indulge* or *not to indulge*. That really is the question, and surprisingly, the answer is based on what you have already eaten *or* what you will be eating in the near future:

Should I Indulge?

- Have I already indulged in a treat-type item (e.g., candy bar, cookies, soda, etc.) or meal less than two hours ago?

  → If *yes*, then definitely pass—*you are probably just eating for recreation*;
  → If *no*, then **think long and hard** to be sure that you **really** want to eat it.

- Will I be eating lunch/dinner in less than an hour?

  → If *yes*, then definitely pass—*it is better to wait*;
  → If *no,* then think **do I really, really want this?** If so, have it; otherwise, don't.

You really have to eat more consciously—where you are only eating foods you absolutely enjoy and/or need for nutrition. When this is the case, enjoy your choices without guilt. Otherwise, save the calories for something more enjoyable. *Make every calorie/indulgence count!*

Eating-Like-You-Have-Some-Sense Strategy #8

Now that we are only eating the foods we *really* love, the next thing we need to do is **master portion control and make good choices when we eat out.** *We need to learn when to say "when."* Believe it or not, this is an important key to losing weight and keeping it off. You remember the bacon cheeseburger I mentioned enjoying in an earlier strategy? Well, the thing I didn't mention is that I always cut it in half before I start eating it. I eat half, and then half goes home for dinner or the next day's lunch/dinner. The same thing for the *Jack Daniel's* ribs and shrimp from *TGI Friday's*—even if I want to eat all of the ribs, shrimp, and fries, *I don't.* I either take half home, or I split the meal with my oldest son. This is not quite a fair split because I *never* get half, maybe a third, but *never* half (*boys are so greedy*). However, this is a good thing because I get enough to enjoy one of my favorite meals, *and* I get full (*remember I am drinking a lot of water too*). So it is a win-win situation for me *and* my son.

In order for any weight loss plan to be successful you have to be able to eat in the real world like you have some sense. You can't exist in a vacuum where you are only eating certain foods or pre-packaged meals, so you need a game plan that allows you to go to restaurants with confidence that you are not going to lose your mind and eat yourself silly. I know this is hard because most of the entrees at our favorite restaurants are too big for the average man, let alone for an average-sized woman. This is especially true as many of us are eating bread before dinner (*often using butter—for some reason, I have never liked butter; it looks like yellow fat*), an appetizer, drinks with the meal (*alcoholic or soda*), and maybe even dessert! **That is way too much eating going on!** Did you know that one meal like this can give us more calories/fat than we should take in for the whole day? Well it can, and if this is what happens **every** time we go to a restaurant, *there is going to be trouble...*

Unfortunately, for too many of us, this is what happens *EVERY* time we go out. I think this is one of the main reasons obesity is almost at epidemic proportions in the United States. I have even heard reports that say that not only are we heavier than people in other countries, but our restaurants also serve the largest portions! I also heard that when U.S. chains open restaurants in other countries they scale down the portion sizes to fit in with the eating habits of those consumers, *who usually are a lot slimmer than we are on average.* Well, since the restaurant owners think we eat more, and they are feeding us more, we have to become our own advocate in cutting back what we eat while still enjoying our favorite restaurants…

So what can you do to fight back? Well, for one thing you can start asking servers at restaurants to cut your entrée portion in half, and put it in a container for you to take home. You can also do this yourself, but you need to do it *BEFORE* you start eating. This is especially ideal for restaurants where you know you will have an appetizer, drinks, and dessert. Examples of meals that you can try this on include:

- A large steak or a full rack of ribs w/mashed potatoes or fries like at *TGI Friday's*;
- Large pasta dishes like lasagna or chicken parmigiana (e.g., Olive Garden, etc.);
- So-called "*Individual*" pizzas, which tend to be big enough for two people (e.g., *Bertucci's, California Pizza Kitchen*, etc.);
- Burgers & fries (e.g., *Sweetwater's, Champ's, Ruby Tuesday's*, etc.);
- Shrimp & fries (e.g., *Applebee's, Red Lobster*, etc.)

You have to come prepared to save at least half of your food for a future meal. It can be saved for dinner or the next day's lunch or dinner, but *never* as a snack for the same day. *Forget all about the concept of a late-night snack made up of leftovers from dinner.* You really don't need that. Instead, let your stomach and digestive organs have the break they so desperately need during the late-night hours. Also, for the rare times you don't want to take food home with you, try to reduce the damage by not having anything before/after your meal (e.g., bread, appetizer, dessert, or drinks), and ask your server to forget the fries/potatoes with your order. If you still need something to go with your entrée, you can substitute steamed vegetables. *Your goal is to only eat as much as you need to get full.* "*Full*," but not stuffed.

Another thing you can do is keep your eyes and ears open when you eat out. I say this because it almost feels like restaurants have an undercover mission to cause us to overeat or be overweight with all of the little ways they try to add extra calories to our meals. One example that comes to mind is when I am in line at *Potbelly's* where I see people getting subs, a big bag of chips, and a soda. You would think that would be enough, yet they are asked if they want a milkshake or cookies along with their order. They even have the nerve to put a butter cookie on the straw for the milkshake! *Who really needs a milkshake or cookies with a lunch like that?* Aside from the handful of us who have been blessed with exceptionally fast metabolisms, professional athletes who train a lot or pregnant women (*I think pregnancy is a blessed state, where enjoying ice cream and milkshakes is a perk*), no one needs this much food for lunch!

Well, since it is not in the best interest of restaurants to change, *we have to.* We can still eat out, but we have to make better decisions on what we eat. Speaking of *Potbelly's*, do you know that I can't taste the difference between their skinny/thin whole-wheat and regular whole-wheat bread, but that simple choice saves a third of the bun's calories. So I get it *every time* I eat there. Also, I say no to the chips, sodas, and offers of cookies and milkshakes EVERY time as well. So a regular *Potbelly's* sub with a piece of fruit and some water is more than enough for lunch when I am eating like I have some sense. I try to do the same thing as I buy Italian BMTs for my youngest son from *Subway.* I ask for two pieces of salami and pepperoni instead of three and one piece of ham instead of two. I also scoop out the extra breading from the bun. *He can't even taste the difference.* Did I mention that I only buy six-inch subs with no oil or mayonnaise, just mustard? The boys split a bag of chips, and I throw in fruit and a box drink or better yet, water, and the meal is a lot more kid-friendly. That is what eating like you have some sense is all about, *making the best choices you can make with the food that you enjoy eating.*

To help you think of ways for you to do the same, here are a few more examples from restaurants where I have learned to *eat and act like I have some sense*:

- *Glory Days*

  What do I eat? ➜ Because I live in a house with men, they tend to gravitate toward sports bars, and this happens to be one of their favorites. This restaurant *used* to have a buffalo chicken salad on their menu that I absolutely love. As it turns out they will still make it *if you ask*, so I ask every time I go there. I get them to glaze the chicken in their Glory sauce. It tastes so good on top of the vegetables. I do not get any cheese or dressing—just the veggies and the chicken. It is so good and filling! For the most part I avoid their appetizers because I can't even eat all of the salad any more. In fact, I give my husband the extra meat from my salad!

- *On The Border*

  What do I eat? ➜ This is a place where you can get into a lot of trouble. Before your meal comes there is already a huge bowl of nachos sitting in front of you. Their queso is phenomenal, so I have to get it. My husband and I split the nachos and the queso, which probably should be the end of the meal based on the fat and calories I am sure it contains. When I first started eating here, I used to order three hard-shell beef tacos after the nachos. However, by the time I got to the third taco, I was absolutely miserable. So I finally talked myself into ordering only two, but after eating two, I was still *too* stuffed. After a while, I finally cut back to one taco ala carte. No sides (*rice or refried beans*), no soda, and definitely no dessert. As always, I drink lots of water. I am pleasantly full after eating this meal, and I *really* enjoy it. I also get a kick out of the looks I get when I only order one taco!

- *Famous Dave's*

  What do I eat? ➜ I try not to get an appetizer here because the entrees are so big. I order a lunch portion (*the dinner portion is huge*) of the fried chicken salad—just the veggies and the chicken. I squirt some of their barbeque sauces on the chicken to give the salad more flavor. My husband and I may also split a small order of ribs, so I eat the salad and one/two ribs. It is so good, and after a few glasses of water, I am as full as I can be. I also buy bottles of their sauce (*my kids love it*) for chicken and pork recipes at home.

- *TGI Friday's*

  What do I eat? ➜ I used to split the *Jack Daniel's* rib and shrimp platter with my oldest son. However, now I let the boys split the platter, and I just order a house salad (*only the vegetables*). I then cut up a few pieces of the sesame chicken from the *Jack Daniel's Sampler* appetizer on it.*Yum!!!!* The boys might also share a couple of their shrimp or ribs with me. With water, this is more than enough and DELICIOUS!

- *Olive Garden*

  What do I eat? ➜ This is the only place where I eat salad with cheese and dressing. I also split a *Create a Sampler* with three choices of mozzarella with my sons. I usually get three mozzarella sticks, which I dip in marinara. If I am alone, I take the extras home to the boys. I also love their breadsticks, so I enjoy the *outside* or the *ends* of **one** dipped in marinara. I only eat the crispy parts of restaurant breads. Can you believe that when I add in an order of calamari, this is a full meal for me and the boys? Salad, cheese, breadsticks, calamari (*they split this*), and *water*—none of us ever leave here stuffed, just pleasantly full. I can be talked into sharing a slice of the lemon crème cake on special occasions (e.g., birthdays, good report cards, visiting guests, etc.). However, the more common dessert for me would be decaf with cream and sugar.

- *Applebee's*

  What do I eat? ➜ I do not eat bread or butter before the meal, but I split an order of cheese sticks with my family. Even if I am alone, I still only eat two or three though. Then I order the boneless buffalo wings and a house salad (*no dressing, cheese, eggs or bacon bits—just the vegetables*). I cut a few pieces of the chicken on top of the salad. The seasoning and sauce on the chicken gives the salad a wonderful flavor. I enjoy the taste, and I leave very full even though I can only eat about three-fourths of it. Roughage is not only healthy, it is also very filling when you drink lots of water with it.

Have you noticed that I tend to gravitate toward restaurants with salads when I eat out? Well I am not very good at making salads at home, so I try to get a lot of them when I eat out. I even pick up a fried chicken salad from *Red Robin* every Friday night for my sons. Minus the fried chicken, I think it is a wonderful thing for boys to *choose* to have a salad for dinner. So we can still eat out, but we may just have to tweak our choices. That is basically what it is all about—*making the healthiest choices you can whenever and wherever you are eating.*

Eating-Like-You-Have-Some-Sense Strategy #9

Whether you are eating at home or in a restaurant, always *eat your fruits and vegetables first* when possible. Fruits and vegetables are wonderful because they are full of vitamins and fiber, which makes them very healthy and very *filling*. Yes, we are back to the nutrition thing again. It is a very small change, but it could lead to noticeable benefits in the long run. Say if you are hungry and you eat your favorite foods first (e.g., a burger, steak, sub, ribs, fries, etc.), by the time you get around to the fruits or vegetables you may already be stuffed from the least healthy and most fattening part of your meal. Also, you will be less likely to want to take half of your entrée home at restaurants. So fill up on the healthiest foods first.

I enforce this with my kids at home. The only required foods at lunch/dinner are fruits and vegetables. I don't care about meat, starches, or bread, but *the fruits/vegetables are a must-have. The kids can't have seconds of their favorite foods until the fruits/vegetables are gone.* Isn't it funny that you never have to force anyone to eat their favorite foods, but many of us leave fruits and vegetables on our plates? *Going forward, this should not be you...* I know you may think it won't make much difference, but it does. As an example, a sandwich goes a long way at lunch when I eat a banana, a pickle, an orange, grapes, or soup *first*. As I mentioned before, my favorite is a peanut butter and jelly on whole-wheat bread (*Healthy Life* is the best), which is very filling. It also helps that I take at least two sips of water after every bite of my sandwich. Another example is at dinner, when I eat my broccoli (*I hate it*) and corn first, I can usually get full with only one biscuit (*with the layers taken out*) and one piece of chicken.

Trust me, eating your fruits and vegetables first can help you feel fuller faster and longer, as well as meet the fruit/vegetable recommendation (*five+/day*) set by most medical experts. Then why aren't we doing it? I think it is because many of us are too busy, lack creativity or have not tried enough fruits/vegetables. I know this is the case for me. This is one of the reasons I periodically buy pre-made fruit bowls from the grocery store that have fruits that we might not normally eat like pineapple, melon, and blueberries. The fruit from these bowls can be eaten throughout the day or with any meals that you might not normally have a fruit/vegetable with (e.g., pizza, sandwiches, quesadillas, etc.). You could also try a pre-made veggie bowl/platter, vegetable soup, or add shots (*I use a one-ounce shot glass*) of various juices (e.g., low-sodium V-8, pomegranate, prune, acai, etc.) to your meals or throughout the day. *Remember, it is all about your health and helping you get fuller faster on foods that add value to your body.*

Eating-Like-You-Have-Some-Sense Strategy #10

If you are a habitual fast-food eater, we have to come up with a plan to slowly wean you off of it or to make what you are buying a healthier meal... I say we should only visit these restaurants once a week at a maximum. However, being a busy sports mom, I know how crazy evening and weekend schedules can get, so some concessions and workarounds can obviously be made... One of the ones I have learned is if you are running late with dinner, everyone is starved, and you pick up fast food, *you do not* **have to** *purchase the side items from the restaurant where you bought the main course.* As an example, say you buy a bucket of chicken from *KFC* or *Popeye's*—do you have to buy coleslaw, red-beans and rice, mashed potatoes w/gravy, fries, and/or biscuits? *No, you do not...* You could just buy the chicken and the biscuits if your family really likes them (*one apiece though*), and serve the leftover green beans (*or any other green vegetable*) from last night's dinner, and make some corn or carrots at home (*minus all of the butter these restaurants tend to cook theirs in*). You don't need all of the fattening sides they offer you. Just say no, and use what you have at home.

Also, if you go to a drive-thru to get your kids a cheeseburger or chicken nuggets from *McDonald's* or *Burger King*, they *do not have to* have fries, especially if they already ate fast-food once during the week. Instead, you can grab their main course, go home and add a green and yellow vegetable, soup or an apple, grapes, applesauce, or a fruit cup to go with it. They can have as much of the fruits and vegetables as they need to get full, and once you add water, I think this is a reasonable dinner for a child. Without the fries and the soda, who minds if the kid wants dessert after dinner? I think our troubles come in when we are eating the burger, the fries, the soda, a dessert from the fast-food restaurant (e.g., apple pie, milkshake, etc.) and then a dessert and other sweetened drinks at home too. This is where excess pounds start creeping up, especially on our children. So I am not suggesting that we cut out all indulgences, just modify some of our choices (a cheeseburger instead of a *Big Mac*), and make some relatively painless trade-offs (*a dessert at home over soda*). I have found that, after the initial argument, even children realize that they are full after eating a meal *they thought* would not be enough.

The same goes for us… We can have a chili dog or burger for lunch or dinner, but substituting the fries or chips with a salad, fruits/veggies, or soup makes it a much healthier meal. As you eat it, be sure to take your time, and enjoy the indulgent item slowly—*do not rush while you are eating.* To slow myself down, I take a few sips of water after each bite. So even though I may eat less than some people at lunch/dinner, I walk away feeling like I had a very enjoyable lunch, and you can too if you mix in healthy things with the not-so-healthy ones. This way you get some of the things that you want, but more of what your body needs. It turns into a win-win all around because you will ultimately wind up consuming less calories and fat than you would otherwise. If in the beginning you find yourself rebelling, just tell yourself what I tell my kids when they want to argue about this, "*Just be thankful that you are getting fast-food that you like!*"**End of discussion.** My rule of thumb for my kids, and what I recommend for you, is that you only have fries and/or soda with meals no more than once a week, *if that.*

Now breakfast may be a different story… *McDonald's* is one place where I *used to* struggle for breakfast, especially when we are on vacation. I love their sausage and egg *McGriddles* (*no cheese*), so I used to order **two** sandwiches. One just never seemed like enough, especially during the winter. I love their hotcakes and syrup as well, so I would also eat one of the hotcakes from my sons' platter. *You know this led to trouble right?* Well after learning the error of my ways, *if* I go to *McDonald's* now, I only eat **one** McGriddle with the **one** hotcake (*with syrup, but no butter*). This is more than enough food for most, especially if we are eating like we have some sense. ***Lesson learned:*** *We never need more than one fast-food sandwich/entree*, which my stomach confirmed once I stopped being so greedy.

The "*only one*" philosophy also extends to burgers (*even if they are on the dollar menu*) and sandwiches. I don't care if you missed breakfast, lunch, or dinner, **never give in to the desire to eat more than one.** Also, **never super-size anything,** and avoid mayonnaise and special sauces. If you must have fries, get a small order. I am thankful to say that for the most part, I have lost all desire to eat fast-food burgers/sandwiches. In fact, on a road trip last year, I let my kids eat at *McDonald's* while I pulled into a park and made a peanut butter and jelly sandwich. However, every once in a while I might eat a Wendy's spicy chicken sandwich (*minus the mayonnaise*) if I have a cold or bug (*for some reason, it settles my stomach*). Also, when fast-food is my only option, you might see me eating a *Great-Biggie* fry from *Wendy's*. I try not to eat this way more than a few times a year. Unfortunately, so many of us are stressed and pressed for time that we can be found in fast-food restaurants on a weekly or a daily basis. **We cannot eat this junk day in and day out**, especially more than once a day—*it is just too unhealthy and too fattening*. It is fine *occasionally*, but if you find yourself at one of these restaurants more than once or twice a week, you will want to rethink your eating habits.

Eating-Like-You-Have-Some-Sense Strategy #11

As you eat normally throughout the day **make as many healthy substitutions as you can without feeling deprived.** As you already know, when we feel deprived, it can lead to rebellion/binge eating. So if you really want a doughnut, have "*a*" doughnut. Who cares about the calories/fat in that one indulgence, especially if you follow it up with healthier choices during the course of the day? *If you really want a candy bar, have one! If you really, really want a slice of cake, have it!* However, be sure that you don't have all of these things on the same day (*unless it is your birthday or a **very** special occasion*). Also, if you indulge in these types of foods, be sure that when you want that afternoon *Coke* you choose water instead to help offset the previous indulgence(s), or cut out a snack that you might normally have in the evening.

These are examples of the trade-offs and concessions you can make so you are able to occasionally enjoy some of your favorite foods/treats. Other examples include if you eat a *McGriddle* or a *Waffle Slam* from *Denny's* for breakfast, you should try to eat a lighter lunch, preferably one you made yourself—*not a bacon cheeseburger and fries from Ruby Tuesday's*. Also, if you had a big lunch at a restaurant, do not add a heavy restaurant dinner on top of it. *Sometimes I have eaten cereal with 1 percent milk for dinner when my lunch was too heavy/filling*. In fact, I would recommend limiting your eating to one restaurant a day unless you are vacation, or it is a rare/special occasion. If you search deep within yourself, you will find that you really are not hungry enough to eat as heavily as you normally would after indulgent snacks or restaurant meals. So **make trade-offs, and stick to them so you can enjoy** *what you want, when you want it and not feel guilty or like you have blown a diet*. *Oh yeah, that's right, we are not on a diet, we are just eating like we have some sense!*

Note: I know people who travel for business may find the advice on restaurants hard to swallow, but it can be done. In fact, when I attended a ten-day conference in Hawaii, I struggled at first because I could not eat cereal with 1 percent milk for breakfast. So for the first few days I had a slice of *Starbucks* iced lemon pound cake (*it is divine*) with water. *Of course that could not continue, so by the third day, I started buying a fruit cup and a bottle of juice*. Because I ate out for lunch, I was usually not hungry enough for dinner at a restaurant. So after a few days of throwing away most of my dinner, I decided to stop eating out for lunch. Instead I found a grocery store and bought, *Wonder Lite* whole-wheat bread, *Welch's* grape jelly (*my favorite*) and chunky peanut butter, *Lay's* kettle cooked jalapeno potato chips, fruit, juice and water. It cost a fortune, but it helped me to only eat one meal a day at a restaurant. I stuck with the fruit cups from *Starbucks* for breakfast and enjoyed one restaurant meal (lunch *or* dinner), and I ate at least one meal in my room. Even though I indulged in way too much *Crunch & Munch*, I still didn't gain any weight because of these concessions and all the walking I did. I know it may be hard at first, but *you can do it too—you just need to be willing and creative*.

Eating-Like-You-Have-Some-Sense Strategy #12

Do you tend to overeat by snacking before dinner or while you are making dinner? I mean polishing off junk-food like *Cheetos*, chips, cookies, crackers, etc? *I ask because I have certainly been there and done that*. If you have too, then maybe **before you leave work to head home or before you start making dinner, you should grab a healthy snack** such as an ounce of walnuts mixed with a small box of raisins and/or sunflower seeds and macadamias (*I mix all four and drink a shot of V-8*) or some fruit. Healthy snacks such as these can leave you feeling calmer and more satisfied as you are cooking dinner or trying to make a healthy dinner choice. So you are less likely to have a fattening snack before dinner.

However, if you cannot/don't want to eat before you start dinner, how about pouring a few ounces of 100 percent juice (e.g., grape, orange, or pomegranate) in a nice glass (e.g., wine, champagne, etc.), and sip it while you cook. The sweetness will help you get over the hump until dinner, and the nice glass will make you feel like you are actually enjoying a treat. In addition to that, you are actually helping to boost your immune system. 100 percent juices are healthy, and many of us calorie-conscious people do not enjoy enough of them. If you have a juicer (*I bought my husband the one by Jack LaLane for Christmas*), it works even better, because you can throw a few fruits or vegetables into it (e.g., grapes, apples, strawberries, carrots, celery, etc.), and you and your family can get some fruits/veggies in before dinner. Again, I do shots of it, but my sons, *even the one who won't eat fruit without force*, drinks it. **Your goal:** Substitute a little something healthy in the place of your usual pre-dinner junk-food or the extra dinner you might ordinarily consume.

Eating-Like-You-Have-Some-Sense Strategy #13

Do not keep or eat food in your car. When you are on a trip, it is OK, but just driving around on a daily basis, it is not. *Of course, there is always room for exceptions.* As I tell you not to eat in your car, I feel I must come totally clean and tell you that there are times you may have seen me with a box of *Crunch & Munch* or a can of *Pringles* in my car, and I am popping one bite after another like I have completely lost my mind. If you have, you can be sure it was the week before/during *a certain monthly event,* or I am struggling to balance the stress of family, home, and career. These are some of the times when I am completely out of control, and I have a strong desire for chocolate, sugar and/or salt. During these times, I may just say *it is what it is,* even if I eat the whole box of *Crunch & Munch* in one sitting, which at times I have.

Why am I telling you this? Well, one reason is because I like to be honest, but also because I think it is important for you to know that we are never going to be perfect. *Everyone has moments where they lose control, and these moments are not deal breakers.* When I lose my mind, I just return to my normal eating habits starting with the next meal. The moment of craziness has passed, and things go back to normal with my eating except for the fact that my usual after-dinner snack is history. These crazy moments are just *temporary* periods where you eat like you don't have any sense, but they don't prevent you from eating like you have some sense for the long-term. *They are just momentary lapses...*

I know some of you may not have the same craving for salt or sugar, but we all have times where we are vulnerable and have a temporary desire to indulge in *something* really bad for us. A lot of times it is caused by a difficult day/period in our lives, and I say you might want to go ahead and make an exception or short-term allowance for this time. As an example, if your husband just left you for a younger woman, I would not look twice at you if I saw you eating a whole box of chocolate *Turtles* or a pint of ice cream in your car. Other examples include if your fiancé left you at the altar, or if you just lost a loved one or a job. In these instances, a little self-pity/emotional eating is completely understandable, especially when followed/accompanied by a good, long cry. *However*, after a few days, *the overindulging must stop*, and you must look within or to someone you trust (e.g., friend, relative, spouse, priest/pastor, counselor, etc.) to help you start putting the pieces back together again and let food return to its proper place—*as a means of nourishment, not as a comforter/friend.*

After you have recovered or made the necessary adjustments, I don't expect to see you eating in the car! Your kids can eat in the car though—*because kids will be kids.* Just bring healthy snacks for them that you won't be tempted to eat (e.g., fruit, string cheese, granola bars, Goldfish, etc.) too. *Just wait until you get home, so you can focus on and control what you are eating!* Eating in the car is usually bad news, especially when it is fast-food. *So don't do it!*

Eating-Like-You-Have-Some-Sense Strategy #14

If you have stayed on track with your eating for breakfast, lunch, and dinner, the only area left to control is how much you are snacking. This is usually one of the hardest areas for us to maintain control over because so many snacks are readily available. For this reason, it is critical that we **find low-fat, low-**

calorie, *high-enjoyment* snacks that we love so we feel rewarded/ indulged. This will help us make it through the day, but more importantly, it should help us make it through the evening without snacking. If I have eaten normally during the day (*not too much pigging out*), I often have a light/small dessert after dinner.

My all-time favorite dessert when I am serious about being as lean as I can be is an orange ice cream bar made by *Giant* (a grocery store chain in the Washington, D.C., area). I used to eat a similar bar by *Pet* called *Dreamsicles* when I was a kid. They have orange sherbet on the outside with ice cream on the inside. They are *soooooooo* good! The best thing is that they are only about eighty calories, with less than five grams of fat. However, another good thing is that it takes you at least five minutes to eat it, so you feel like you are really indulging yourself. Sometimes I have even eaten two. *Why not?* It's only 160 calories, which is almost the equivalent of three *Oreos* or a small bag of chips, but you get a lot more satisfaction and less fat. A frozen fudge bar may be a better alternative for chocoholics like me because it only has 110 calories, it takes longer to eat, and it only has 2.5 grams of fat! Another one of my favorite after-dinner treats is a few pieces of caramel as I drink from my mug of ice water. It is so rich and sweet that I feel really indulged and satisfied afterward.

I mention after-dinner snacking because that is an area that trips many of us up, but the snacking you do during the day is also a potential area for disaster. For this reason, you will also need to *find healthy or not-so-healthy snacks that you can indulge in during the day*, which you can eat in moderation. As I mentioned before, I cannot be trusted to eat just three or four *Oreos, Keebler Fudge Covered Graham Crackers* or *Reese's Miniature Peanut Butter Cups*, so I just don't buy them as regular treats anymore. Everyone has a food(s) that they cannot be trusted with—for some it could be ice cream, cheese, cookies, chips, cake, etc… It is up to you to find out what your weakness is, and avoid it until you can eat that food in moderation. In the meantime, find enjoyable substitutes because you are going to want to snack. *So find your backup snacks in advance (e.g., Dreamsicles,* caramel, low-fat popcorn, etc.). If you are caught unprepared, the tendency to overindulge in high-fat, high-calorie foods is more likely—I call this "*showing out.*" However, the question I reluctantly ask myself when I have been showing out is, "*Do I want to be a size 6, or do I want to eat cookies?*" Hmmmm?

After much thought and agonizing, I accept the fact that *I want to be a size 6*, so I have to make the necessary adjustments to get myself back under control. So, what size/weight do you want to be, and what adjustments are you prepared to make to get/stay there? To get/stay wherever you decide you want to be requires that you be prepared with reasonable snacks at all times *for you and your family.* Along with this, here are a few additional tips to help you:

1. A regular-sized candy bar is plenty! Don't buy jumbo size candy bars unless it a special occasion. Also, you don't need a candy bar every day— *these should be rare treats.*
2. If you choose to eat chips, *do not eat them from a bag.* Eating from a bag does not allow you to *see* how much you are eating, but you need to *see* what you are eating so you can monitor portion sizes. Chips are not necessarily bad *(well they are kind of),* but eating too many of them can be. So don't eat them every day—*they should also be rare treats.*
3. Do not keep cookies in a cookie jar at your house. I know it looks so decorative and welcoming when you see this on television or in someone else's house, but if you/your kids don't have control in this area, you might want to keep something else in the jar—*maybe seashells or marbles!* It's not that you have to eliminate carbs, you just need to reduce the number of carbs you are snacking on (e.g., cake, doughnuts, and crackers). **That means stop eating so many doggone cookies!** We have lost our minds with the amount of unconscious eating we do with these types of junk-food. *So it is time to stop.*

One way that you can limit the amount of junk-food you eat is by increasing your fruit intake. I know I keep going back to the fruit thing, but the natural sugar in it can help you get your sweet tooth under control *once you are really committed to make a change.* Until you are really ready, start off slowly, and get you/your family exposed to more fruits by bringing home one new fruit a week (e.g., kiwi, pomegranate, mango, etc.). Some you will like, some you won't, but the more you try, the more you will like. The end result will be that you will eat more fruit, and you will become healthier and slimmer as some of the junk-foods you currently eat are replaced by healthier choices. It's funny that we may enjoy eating certain fruits, but they are not the first thing we usually think of grabbing when we are hungry for a snack. *This needs to change.* Sometimes before I grab a sweet treat, I try a piece of fruit to see if it will satisfy my craving (e.g., an orange or a banana before a candy bar, etc.). Many times it does not work, but *sometimes* it is enough to make me forget all about the junk-food. So my suggestion is to stock up on fruits that you like, as well as low-fat treats that you enjoy (e.g., small cups of yogurt, applesauce, pretzels, gingersnaps, popcorn, graham crackers, cereal with low-fat milk, frozen fruit bars, individual sherbet cups, etc.). This should make it easier for you to make wise choices when it is time to snack. *You have to be prepared if you are going to do succeed.*

Eating-Like-You-Have-Some-Sense Strategy #15
Look for signals that your body is giving you regarding what/ how much you are eating. I learned to do this over a period of years through trial and error, *mostly error*. Say if I had pastries/doughnuts and coffee (*loaded with sugar*) for breakfast, I usually felt a little weird if I ate peanut butter and jelly for lunch. The sweet taste of the jelly at lunch is not as enjoyable after I have had sweets for breakfast. In fact, I feel queasy when I eat sweets back to back or have too many at once, especially when I am not drinking lots of water with them. It took a few years for me to finally accept this, but now that I have, the knowledge helps me decide what I will/will not eat on a given day.

Other signals I learned to listen to were the recurring heartburn and twinges in my diaphragm (*started as I approached forty*) that occurred when I combined chocolate, tomato sauce, and/or grease with caffeinated drinks. I ignored the symptoms for a while and continued to eat as I pleased; however, after three trips to the doctor with symptoms that made them think that either I had a blood clot or something was wrong with my pancreas or heart, I started to listen. It was a scary and costly lesson—*I had to have blood work, an EKG, an ECG*, and at the last visit the doctors were even searching online for clues to find out what was wrong with me! After all of the tests confirmed that nothing major was wrong, the next question was ALWAYS, "*What did you eat before you noticed the symptoms,*

Mrs. Gray?"It wasn't obvious to me when I went to the doctor that it was always the same types of food, but of course when they asked, I could then think back to a specific incident where I overindulged in the foods I mentioned.

Well, after having to take *Nexium* **and** *Prilosec* a few times, I finally got it. So now I only drink decaf, which really is not even a big deal because caffeine usually doesn't even help to keep me awake (*the only exception is the Red Bull I drink on Fridays, but many times I still take a nap first*)! As long as I respect the new boundaries my body has set for me (*avoiding the food combinations I mentioned*), I am no longer plagued with those troubling symptoms. So many times our bodies give us clues as to how we should modify our eating, but a lot of times we are not listening to the hints that can often make us feel better. Think of the times where you may notice that your "*bathroom habits*" are not as normal / *regular* as they usual are, your body is often telling you to eat more fiber, more salads, more fruits and vegetables, and / or to drink more water. We usually take the cues to mean we need medicine from the drug store—sometimes *maybe*—but many times no; **we just need to balance our eating better.**

Eating-Like-You-Have-Some-Sense Strategy #16

Do not eat in front of the television. Until you have your eating impulses under control, you should not eat while you are distracted. It is hard enough for you to realize that you are full and to stop eating when you are just sitting at the table focusing on the act of eating, but it is infinitely harder to do this when you are being entertained. I think you should have a significant amount of time eating and acting like you have some sense under your belt before you even think about plopping down in front of the TV with your plate. We are all more likely to eat mindlessly or overeat when we do this. So this should not be our normal way of eating meals, especially dinner.

Even when you get to the point where you feel comfortable enough to do this (*I must admit that I eat pizza in front of the TV on Friday nights*), if you struggle with after-dinner snacking, you may want to turn off the TV during food commercials. Some of those commercials make overindulging look like it is the best thing in the world, and they often make you think that everyone else in the world is eating this way. Well, much of the world is not, and many of those who have struggle with their weight. The commercials also make us feel that we deserve to overeat but, except for the rare occasion, this is usually not true. *So don't believe the hype, and turn that TV off until you are done eating.*

Eating-Like-You-Have-Some-Sense Strategy #17
Limit your alcohol intake, especially when it comes to the large, fancy drinks in restaurants and bars. As I mentioned before I stopped drinking alcohol over fifteen years ago, and I have since come to view it as a big, fat waste of calories for me personally. However, I read an article a few years ago called *To Drink or Not to Drink* by Amy Paturel, MS, MPH, on *AOL* under *AOL Diet & Fitness,* which let me know that I may not be so far off base. The author of the article warned that if we are not careful a lot of the large, fruity, slushy drinks women tend to love, could add up to a whole lot of extra calories— *possibly thousands.* In the article, Tara Gidus, MS, RD, of the American Dietetic Association, also pointed out that drinking cocktails does not make us feel as full as we would if we ate food with a similar caloric value. So, basically they can be fattening, but usually are not very filling, so the tendency is to keep drinking out of taste/thirst. *How many of you know that this can certainly lead to trouble if you go out socializing or drinking on a regular basis?*

Well, according to the article you may want to be especially careful with daiquiris, Pina Coladas, Long Island Ice Tea, mixers, and coolers. You'd be lucky to find any of these drinks under two hundred calories, and some may even have more than five hundred calories! Still, having *one* of these drinks is not a bad thing. However, if you are honest, you know they are like potato chips—*most people can't stop at one.* Even though *most* should… Maybe it would help if we thought of these drinks as alcoholic desserts, *which they are.* So as with sobriety and eating in general, moderation is definitely the key, so *you must drink like you have some sense as well.*

Don't get me wrong, *I am not suggesting that you stop drinking like I did. That is a personal choice I made, but it has nothing to do with you.* However, I would suggest that you only indulge in one of these drinks when you are out with friends, especially if weight is an issue for you, and/or you will be eating quite a bit (e.g., bread, appetizer, etc.). *Would it kill you to drink a few glasses of water before and after your drink, nurse your drink a bit once you get it, and maybe drink a cup of coffee afterward?* This one choice could save you hundreds of calories, especially as you may be less likely to overeat when your judgment is not impaired by drinking. Either way, you will definitely want to choose your drinks more carefully…

Eating-Like-You-Have-Some-Sense Strategy #18

No late-night eating! Trust me, nothing good comes from eating at night, especially when you have already had breakfast, lunch, dinner, and snacks. Let's face it, most times you are not even hungry. You are usually just eating to be eating, and after a long, busy/stressful day, *you could pack on a lot of extra calories if you are not careful.* I am not even going to try to make you think that I am so beyond this because I am not. I completely understand that after a long hard day, especially after working, cooking, cleaning, putting kids to bed, we often feel like we deserve a treat. For me, it used to be chocolate, cookies, or ice cream, but when I got serious (*see Wake-up Call #3, Chapter 3*), I *DECIDED* that I would no longer eat after 9:00 p.m. I wanted to say 8:00, but I had to be realistic as I tried to get used to not eating at night.

Because old habits die hard, I had to come up with some satisfying alternatives to my late-night eating and make some major behavior modifications. So after some thought, I came up with a few "treats" that I could enjoy without eating. One of these is a tall glass of "sweet" tea. Growing up in Georgia, I must say I can make some really good sweet tea. I boil a pot of water, and steep four bags of *Bigelow* green tea and three bags of *Lipton* tea together. Green tea has many health benefits, and I have even heard it is supposed to help speed up the metabolism—*of course I can't confirm that.* I avoid bottled teas because I don't believe they offer the same antioxidant benefit, they are too large, and they probably have more calories than mine has. My other nighttime drinks include: a tall glass of *Welch's* grape juice with ice and a shot of water; a tall glass of ice cold 1 percent milk with a heaping tablespoon of *Nestle Quick* chocolate mix (the powder), or coffee with cream and sugar. *Only one glass/cup though*, and for the rest of the night I drink ice water from my mug. Water is so good when it is cold, and it helps keep you feeling satisfied if you eat normally during the day (*no skipped meals*).

When I first started this practice, I struggled at first, but within a few months, I decided to change the cutoff time from 9:00 to 8:00. To take my mind off eating, I started doing positive things with my time in the evening—writing, reading, working on my laptop, exercising, or hanging out with my husband. The secret was to find something enjoyable to do, get my tea, milk, or coffee, and go upstairs—*no hanging out in the kitchen.* This is a time when I might work on creative activities that I enjoy. It does not really matter what you do (e.g., knitting, reading, folding clothes, walking on the treadmill, or watching television, etc.) as long as you find it interesting or distracting. It is pretty hard to eat chips or ice cream while you are knitting or walking. If you can't find anything that you really want to do, just *GO TO BED!*

Keep reminding yourself that nothing good comes from eating after 8:00 p.m. The only things I have ever gotten from it are love handles, a little extra fat on my arms/back, and a noticeable rubbing of my thighs! So do whatever you have to do to change your habits. For example, do not keep food of any kind in your bedroom, and try not to eat there except on very rare occasions. Also, until you are strong enough, turn the volume down as you watch food commercials, or look away/leave the room. Until you get your late-night snacking under control, food commercials should be off-limits. *Do you think it is healthy for recovering alcoholics to watch beer/liquor commercials?* No, it is not, because it can lead to them falling off the wagon. So longingly watching food commercials could cause you to fall off the wagon—*where you eat when you are not hungry* and *eat like you don't have any sense.* So again, whatever you need to do to limit eating after dinner is a worthwhile effort in the long run.

I think this one strategy helps to speed up my weight loss efforts the most because it gives my body almost twelve hours between dinner and breakfast to digest food and burn calories. Calories taken in late in the evening, especially close to bedtime, are usually stored as fat unless you have an unusually fast metabolism or you work out a lot. If you do not, you should avoid eating less than three hours before bedtime. Of course there will be times when you make the occasional exception (e.g., parties, anniversary celebrations, vacations, etc.). However, to get and keep extra pounds off, the slipping and exceptions should be very, very rare. For me, the best thing about not eating at night is that it keeps my weight from slipping beyond five to six pounds during times when I am eating more and exercising less (*likely to happen in the winter*). So it is not as hard to get back where I need to be.

When we get beyond ten or fifteen pounds of our desired weight, it feels almost impossible, if not infinitely harder, to get back on track. So I think this tip can definitely help us keep our weight within a more maintainable range because it helps cut our snacking and emotional eating significantly. Sometimes my husband offers me food when he is eating late at night, and he jokingly asks, "*Why don't you eat something?*" Even though I am often tempted, I usually say, "*I'll live—I can make it until breakfast.*" Then I go upstairs. A few times I have even told him when he is trying to eat big meals late at night, "*Go to bed, you'll live. You can certainly wait until morning.*" It is true; we will not starve to death during the night if we forego the so-called *midnight snack*. You will probably also sleep better! **Note:** If you are a diabetic or have health conditions that require you to eat, by all means get a light, sensible snack as your physician suggests. However for those who don't, just get some ice water, and *take your butt back to bed!* If you still can't sleep, try writing down a list of goals/dreams you would like to accomplish, as well as the things you can do to help make them happen.

Emergency Situation Tips: What if for some reason you missed dinner, it is after your eating curfew, and you are starving? You could wait until the morning and just enjoy your one nighttime snack (e.g., milk, juice, etc.), remembering that you will live. I have done this before, but it requires skipping a meal, which is never a good thing. So a nice compromise might be to have cereal (e.g., *Raisin Bran*, *Cheerios*, etc.) and 1 percent milk instead of making a big dinner or grabbing fast-food. It is filling, low in fat, full of fiber, calcium, and iron, and it tastes good. There are other quick choices you could make such as: soup, fruit and a sandwich (e.g., a BLT, grilled cheese, tuna fish, etc.); soup and crackers, or a salad dressed up with leftover meat. The goal is to **eat light at night.** If your stomach growls afterward just have your nighttime drink, drink plenty of water, and think how good it will feel when you reach your goal weight! Then GO TO BED!!!!!!! Seven to eight hours of sleep will help your health more than any late-night snack or doctor's pill ever could. *Remember, late-night hours are for sleeping not eating!*

Eating-Like-You-Have-Some-Sense Strategy #19

In addition to my recommendation that you avoid late-night eating, I must also say *do not get in the bed after eating if possible (especially if you had a heavy meal)*—*not to watch TV, read, or to go to sleep.* **You should try to move around at least a few hours after eating** (e.g., doing housework, shopping, walking, etc.). This is one of the reasons why, whether I work out during the day or night, I always want to take a walk after dinner. It just makes me feel better, especially if I ate a heavier meal than I should have. I bet it will make you feel better too. Even if your mobility is limited, *just do whatever you can do.* Moving, *especially after eating*, helps keep our metabolisms revved up and *burning.* However, *when we sit or sleep on food, it usually doesn't get burned, it is more likely to get stored as fat.*

I think of the food that we sleep or lie down on as *the life-support to our love handles.* Our goal is to cut off their food supply so they have no reason to *hang* around. This is one of the reasons I work so hard not to eat in the evenings—*it is the perfect time for your body to burn off some of the extra fat that is just hanging around and taking up space.* So in the evenings be selective about what you eat, and then **keep it moving after you eat, any way you can.**

Eating-Like-You-Have-Some-Sense Strategy #20

For the most part I don't want you to listen to unsolicited comments on your weight. However, *listening to some (not all) people's comments can be good, especially when it relates to your eating habits.* Remember in Wake-up Call #2 my mother said, *"You need to lay off of that old chocolate,"* and my stepdaughter said, *"You must really be hungry,"* as I ate my second big bowl of *Captain Crunch?* Well although I didn't want to listen, *they were right!* I did need to *lay off of that old chocolate,* and *I wasn't hungry enough for that second bowl of cereal!* Looking back, I am so glad that I listened and made the necessary changes because they were critical steps that helped me to lose the rest of my baby weight.

Another example of this happened a few years ago when I worked for *Sprint.* I had developed a *habit* where I indulged in doughnuts *every* Friday for breakfast. I would buy a bag of *Krispy Kreme* mini crullers or a box of doughnuts (e.g., chocolate, glazed, powdered, etc.). I would have coffee with either five or six mini crullers or *three* regular-sized doughnuts. Then I would leave the rest in the kitchen for my co-workers. I never looked at the number of calories or fat information on the package because *I didn't even want to know.* Well I should have since I was also drinking soda in the afternoon at that time (*my "excuse" was that the caffeine might help increase the effectiveness of the Tylenol Sinus I was taking*), which is usually a no-no for me. However, when you find yourself in an office setting and *you really don't want to be*, you often find yourself coming up with ways/excuses/crutches to help you get through the day.

Well, imagine my annoyance as I put a bag of leftover mini crullers in the kitchen, and a guy that walked in to have one decided that he would read and share the nutritional information on the back of the bag. **Who asked him to do that?** I kept saying, *"Man, I don't even want to know..."* He could have had as many of them as he wanted, but for him to give me information that I didn't want to hear was going too far! Much to my dismay, he told me how much fat, cholesterol, and calories those sinful things had. Although I did not want to hear what he was saying, it spoke to me as much as it annoyed me. Still I tried to explain away the significant caloric/fat indulgence by saying that I only did it on Fridays, but he asked, *"Wouldn't it be easier to reach your beach weight loss goal if you stopped eating these?"* Of course I had shared that I wanted to lose five pounds before going to the beach, and *he remembered!*

Just like when my mother and stepdaughter made their comments, I listened grudgingly, and I don't think I have had mini crullers since! This is also kind of interesting because during this same period, I also remember my husband once jokingly asked, *"How many cookies are you going to eat?"* I think I must have bought cookies and overindulged to the point where he didn't get any. The final straw came after he made me get on our scale to make sure that it was working properly (*I don't like scales*). *Somehow* two pounds had "mysteriously" crept on even though I had been exercising more regularly. This was less than a month from our beach trip so, based on the comments of the guy at work *and my husband*, I finally realized that I had to nip some bad habits in the bud if I was going to get back on track and reach my goal.

So I switched to biscotti (110 calories instead of 1,000+ calories) with coffee on Fridays. Also, I started having a cup of green/*Lipton* tea with my sinus medicine instead of soda. Guess what? It worked the same, and it is a much healthier choice. I also stopped buying cookies *again*, and put the "*8:00 p.m. eating rule*" back in effect after a few too many late-night dinner violations. This coupled with playing tennis with my sons and running a few laps around the track afterward helped me reach my *two-piece-ready* goal just in time for the trip. *I am so glad I listened!* So sometimes we may need to consider the annoying comments directed our way—not the insulting or demeaning ones—but the ones that could be divinely orchestrated.

Eating-Like-You-Have-Some-Sense Strategy #21

Sometimes when we are tempted to binge/eat unhealthy snacks, unorthodox methods may be required. One of the methods that *sometimes* works for me is to **prolong the decision to eat and distract yourself for at least fifteen minutes.** Meditate or do whatever else you can think of while you wait. It doesn't matter *what* you do, but you need to create a delay. I came up with this idea one day as I was sitting at my desk in the late afternoon. I decided to have a *Krispy Kreme* mini cruller with my water. IT WAS *SO* GOOD, *so* I decided to have one more… I tried to remind myself that it was *Fun Food Friday*, and I was having pizza that night, but that did not stop me from wanting another one. So I had one more, and it was so light and sweet, and with the water it was truly divine! *I had to have another one.* The taste in my mouth was absolutely incredible. *Would it really be so bad if I ate the rest of the bag (it was leftover from breakfast)?* Once I had this thought *I knew I was in trouble!*

I wasn't even hungry, and even if I were, I should have been making healthier choices in light of my dinner plans. As a result, I decided to put the bag down, and I closed my eyes, sat still and breathed deeply while I *slowly* counted to a hundred (not a fast one-two-three-four, but more like one------two-------three --------four). I was trying desperately to stall until I could eat like I had some sense again. *After reaching one hundred, I still wanted the rest of the crullers.* So I had a few sips of water, and then I left my desk to go do something else. By the time I came back to my desk, the *snack attack* had passed, so I was able to resist the temptation to eat possibly four or five more crullers. I then almost ran to put the bag back in the kitchen for others to enjoy, and I waited until dinner before eating anything else. So the lesson I learned is that when you see your eating is spiraling out of control, *take a time-out* to breathe and count to one hundred even if you have to go somewhere where there is no food. *Oh yeah, I also learned not to keep doughnuts in my desk!*

Eating-Like-You-Have-Some-Sense Strategy #22

Because excessive snacking is usually the weakest link for anyone who is struggling to lose or maintain their weight (*I know it is mine*), one more tip on getting this area under control is needed: **Put a limit on your non-healthy snacking.** I know this is much easier said than done, but *it must be done!* Too many of us are snacking after breakfast (*pastries, candy, etc.*), snacking after lunch (*candy, cookies, chips, soda, etc.*), and snacking after dinner (*cookies, chips, soda, beer, etc.*). *There is only so much snacking that should be done in a day,* and we are going way over that limit in many of these examples. Do we really need to indulge in junk-food after *every* meal?

No we do not! I really believe that advertisers and food manufacturers have brainwashed us (*via commercials*) into thinking that unhealthy snacking throughout the day is not only acceptable, but it is a normal way to eat and drink. They have successfully reshaped the eating/drinking habits of generations of consumers, and unless we start acting and raising our kids differently, obesity could become a generational curse. The eating/drinking habits of parents usually become the habits of their children and so on. I think this is one of the main reasons the obesity rates continue to rise. So I want to go on record as saying that *junk-food should only represent a small percentage of our daily diet* because after all, *it is junk*—it provides us with no real nutritional value, usually just empty calories.

For this reason, we need to practice saying no to junk-food after at least one of our three meals on a regular basis. As an example, I would replace your usual mid-morning and mid-afternoon snacks with something healthy (e.g., a banana, orange, yogurt, nuts, etc.). However, if you can't part with your afternoon candy bar, chips, or soda, maybe you could make changes to your mid-morning and after-dinner snacks instead? Remember how I told you that I used to eat a chocolate doughnut every night when I was at my skinniest weight? Well, during the times I did this, I only ate a banana for my mid-morning snack, and if I ate a snack in the afternoon, it was a pack of crackers/cookies from the vending machine, but that was it—a six-pack of *Swiss* cookies and one chocolate doughnut. *Very satisfying*, but not excessive. I only chose to eat what I absolutely had to have. I said *no* to the rest. *You should do the same.*

The secret to doing this, *getting your snacking under control,* lies in your ability to make concessions. You have to be willing to identify what snacks you are willing to live without and *the ones you aren't.* Then make concessions or trade-offs to make room for the ones you can't live without, and *stop buying/eating the snacks you can live without.* You can't have it both ways *and* lose or keep the weight off unless you are willing to majorly step up the exercise, which few of us are willing to do. So I would just focus on eliminating the snacks that you can live without. You will be surprised that there are more than you think, and as you slowly replace them with healthier choices or forego them altogether, you will notice that your desire for them will diminish. The other thing you will notice is that the numbers on the scale will start moving in the right direction. *However, it is up to you and the choices you make.*

Eating-Like-You-Have-Some-Sense Strategy #23

Journal Smournal. Keeping a food journal, where you write down everything you eat in a day, works for some people, and if it works for you, I say more power to you—keep doing whatever works. *However, I never do it and I don't recommend it.* This is mainly because it takes more time than I want to devote to such a task, and it puts too much focus on food, making it seem that all of your life/thoughts revolve around food. In my opinion, the thought and effort required to maintain a food journal only adds to the whole *what-are-we-going-to-eat* and *what-are-we-going-to-drink* next obsession. I could be wrong, *but to me,* it seems obsessive. I know it helps you keep a written record of what you have eaten *when you are trying to delude yourself,* but I don't see this practice as a part of the long-term solution.

Even though I am against food journals, *I am not against journaling.* In fact, I think a better alternative to journaling about what you eat or drink would be to journal your thoughts and feelings *before and after* you eat or drink. I say this because most of the times when we carry extra weight, there are emotional issues that we may not be dealing with (*See Chapter 4 for more on this*). If there are emotional issues, having a written record of the thoughts and feelings that led you to eat in the first place and how you felt afterward, may give you the ammunition you need to address those feelings once and for all. *So instead of focusing on what you are eating (a symptom), focus on your thoughts/ feelings ("why" you are eating).* Once you know *why* you are overeating and deal with it, *you will eat less.*

Eating-Like-You-Have-Some-Sense Strategy #24

As you eat and act like you have some sense, there is one thing I cannot say enough: *Eating healthier and maintaining your weight is a step-by-step, day-by-day process, not an all-or-nothing proposition.* If you don't make the best choices today or this week, *it is not the end of the world.* So you don't have to beat yourself up or try to punish yourself by eating very little or working out twice as hard the next day. Just resume your *eating-like-you-have-some sense* routine the next day or whenever you get back from vacation, whatever the case may be. Remember, it is the consistent/chronic overeating and inactivity that packs on extra pounds. *Not the occasional slip-ups.* As a result, if you consistently eat like you have some sense and stay active, it will be easier to reach and maintain a healthy weight.

For this reason, I say slip-ups are definitely allowed *and expected* because *WE ARE HUMAN.* Sometimes we will fall off the wagon or take temporary breaks from our normal patterns (e.g., Thanksgiving, Christmas, vacations, birthdays, etc.); that's life. However, as long as we get back on track as soon as possible, we can stay on target for our weight loss/maintenance goals, *whatever they are.* **Remember, tomorrow is a new day. So if you have messed up on any of these strategies, it is OK.** It does not mean you are a failure or that you will never lose the weight. All it means is that you had a bad day or period. *So acknowledge it.* Learn from it, and do what you know to do tomorrow and the day after.

Eating-Like-You-Have-Some-Sense Strategy #25

Finally, if we want to achieve or maintain a healthier weight, it is well within our reach. However, as you DECIDE to get serious and go for it, *don't be tempted to take unhealthy shortcuts such as diet pills, meal replacement shakes, colon cleanses, or unrealistic low-calorie diets that you can't follow for the long-term.* Ultimately, these types of diets or plans will leave you in the same boat as before, *or worse*, and many times with a slower metabolism than you had before you started. Starving yourself is not only unhealthy, but it can also have a reverse effect on your metabolism.

When you drastically reduce your caloric intake, your body essentially says, *"There is a crisis or a food shortage, so we need to slow down and conserve calories so we don't starve to death."* Sure you may lose some weight, but when you start eating normally again, with this slower metabolism, you will probably gain the weight back faster and maybe even more of it! This is usually what happens when people come off of liquid diets or plans where they buy pre-made meals/shakes from a company. **Bottom line:** There are no shortcuts—*you have to learn how to prepare, select, and eat real food on your own. Jenny Craig, Nutrisystem,* and *Weight Watchers* can't do it for you, although they may be able to help you get the ball rolling. *However, you are the only one who can change your lifestyle to include good eating and exercise habits that YOU can live with for a lifetime.* And, let's face it, that's what this is all about—a weight loss/maintenance plan that is safe and flexible enough to be used for a lifetime. So always remember: *Whatever you do to lose weight, you must be prepared to do that for the rest of your life if you are to be successful.* **NO SHORTCUTS!**

Tying It All Together

Believe it or not I *try* to utilize each and every one of these strategies in my daily efforts to eat *and* act like I have some sense. Of course, I can't get my mind and body to cooperate *every* day or even every week, so I just take it day by day. I think that is the most important thing—that *you just keep moving forward, no matter what happened yesterday or last week.* For the most part, these strategies have become a way of life for me, so I have more days where I am happily "on the wagon" than I have off. If anyone were to ask me what is my secret for losing weight and keeping it off, the answer would definitely be a mixture of the time-tested strategies I just shared with you. These strategies provide the framework that keeps me from straying too far, and they serve as reminders to help me do what I know to do over the long-term. Guess what else? The more strategies I practice consistently, the easier it is for me to comfortably fit in my skinny jeans and proudly sport my favorite bikini without major effort.

However, when I stumble or stray too far from these strategies (e.g., eating after 8:00 p.m. too often, indulging in too much chocolate, eating out for lunch too many times in a week, etc.), my skinny jeans tend not to be as comfortable, and I am not as proud *or* as comfortable in that bikini. When this happens, I usually ask myself, "*What were you thinking? You know better!*" Then I run back to my arsenal of *eat-like-you-have-some-sense* strategies to get back on track. This is why I don't follow the latest diet crazes or buy new diet books because *diets don't work over time.* Maybe they have for you, but chances are *if you are reading this book, I suspect they haven't.* I think diets are just quick fixes that leave you looking for something new to try when they fail. On the other hand, my plan for *eating like you have some sense is not a diet; it is a way of life.* So just as you have to remind yourself to maintain good habits such as getting a good night's sleep, getting a physical, and taking your vitamins, you may also have to occasionally remind yourself to follow these lifestyle strategies as well.

Once these strategies become a way of life, you will definitely be on your way back to wearing your skinny jeans *and* staying in them. I tell you, they have worked for me over the past twenty years—from college to kids, from being a working wife/mother to being middle-aged (ugh!). So it can be done, but your results will be based on *your* commitment *and* consistency. Trust me, you will look *and* feel better, and you will find that a lifestyle change works so much better than any diet ever could. *Come on, what have you got to lose other than weight?*

~

Chapter 9

R e a d j u s t & R e f i n e
Y o u r H a b i t s
(S t e p 7)

Wow, are you still with me? I know I have been long-winded, but I wanted to tell you **EVERYTHING** that has helped me to lose weight and keep it off. Losing weight and keeping it off is not simple, **but it is possible.** I know because I have done it and continue to do it year after year, and the jeans/bikini that still fit are my rewards. Sure, some habits are periodically readjusted and refined, but you can still eat the foods you enjoy while doing it. It really is a process of *eating and acting like you have some sense,* which means getting your emotions and mind under control, eating moderately and making better choices, and moving/exercising above and beyond what you have been doing. As you do this, two things will happen:

1) Either you will start to lose weight *slowly but surely*; or
2) The pattern of weight gain you may have had going on will slow down or stop altogether.

Number one is the best case scenario; however, the importance of not gaining any more weight should not be minimized—let's call this "weight stabilization." Even if you aren't losing weight right away, you certainly don't want to gain any more, so weight stabilization is very important.

Once your weight is stabilized you can successfully move forward, and get beyond the *one-step-forward-two-steps-back* rut you may have been stuck in. This is a very pivotal phase where you can either form counterproductive habits, or *you can propel forward, and just do it!* **I want you to just do it!** *This is your time! The time is now! The weight can be lost* **and** *kept off,* **and you can do it!** So now is not the time to let little habits cause you to go backwards. Here is an example for you to consider: Say your weight has stabilized, and you decide to start drinking a twenty-ounce soda every day at work when you had been drinking water. *This is one of the few times you will hear me talking about calories...* So that's five sodas a week for four weeks (*approximately* twenty *workdays a month*). That's twenty twenty-ounce sodas at 233 calories each, which adds 4,667 extra calories a month. *It adds up doesn't it?* There are 3,500 calories in a pound of fat, so if you did this for a year, and nothing else changed, **you could gain 1.3 pounds per month or 16 extra pounds per year!** A twenty-ounce soda seems harmless enough, and it is by itself, but what you do consistently, *your habits,* truly make or break your weight loss efforts. So replacing that one drink with water can get you in a holding pattern, where your weight is stabilized and you are on the path to actual weight loss.

Developing a Plan for Issue Resolution

Why do you think I used the soda example? Because it is a habit I have personally battled. Winning little battles like this can help us win the overall battle of the bulge. *However, you can't win battles that you don't acknowledge and work to change.* My battle with soda seemed harmless because I would only drink it at work. I loved the way it tasted when it was ice cold, with crushed ice in a Styrofoam cup. So *every day* at 3:00 I would go to the vending area to chat and enjoy *a Coke and a smile.* It seemed *harmless* enough, but with the other snacking I was doing (mini crullers *every* Friday), this *habit* became a **noticeable** issue—*about five pounds* **worth.** Just as with good habits, small changes can add up to a lot over time...

However, once you realize your weight is out of a healthy range (*you can tell by the way your clothes are fitting*) or it is not headed in a good direction, you need to get on a scale and "own the number." I don't get on the scale every day, but I do when I need to *face the music* so I'll be motivated to do what I need to do. I use the scale to help determine how far off course I am. *I can tell when there is a problem because I am usually scared to get on the thing!* Although there are times when we really need to know, most of us don't need to know *every* day. A fluctuation of a few pounds is not cause for alarm, but you want to be able to jump on a situation before you have more than a ten-pound increase. Once you "own the number" and **DECIDE** that you want to do something about it, you have the motivation to readjust/refine.

We always think we have to do something dramatic and excessive to see results, but not gaining another pound based on making a different choice and leaving everything else the same can make a big difference. You saw the significant difference that just cutting out an afternoon soda could make, and *I am doing quite nicely without it, thank you very much!* I bet there are items you can live without as well (e.g., pre-dinner bread, afternoon *Doritos*, extra helpings of mashed potatoes, etc.). Over a day or a week this may not add up to much, but over the course of a month or year, these types of changes can mean the difference between staying the same size *or* needing a larger size each year. I must tell you that it is a wonderful blessing and a treat to try on the same jeans or skirt from a previous year, and they fit exactly the same as they did the year before—*even if you don't want to wear them again*, to be able to wear them *if you want* is a beautiful thing. It is also a beautiful thing when you can keep your body looking relatively lean, and you don't look or feel your particular age. I know most people don't usually realize I am forty-three, and I usually don't feel it *as long as I keep my weight under control...*

Getting To the Size You Want & Staying There

So there you have it. I have given as many tips as I can think of to get you on the path to losing weight and keeping it off. However, I thought I would leave you with my top ten list of things that will help you get to the size you want *and stay there* year after year:

1. Drink WATER at least 90 percent of the time.
2. Do not skip meals, and be sure to eat fruits, vegetables, and whole-grains *every* day.
3. Limit fast-food and processed foods (*e.g., fries, hot dogs, Steak-Ums, etc.*).

4. Only eat foods you *REALLY ENJOY*—if it is just OK, ***don't eat it.***
5. Don't keep snacks in your house that you can't eat in moderation, and *snack with care.*
6. Try not to eat after 8:00 p.m. (*this is when most emotional eating occurs*).
7. Walk instead of driving when possible, and take the stairs/move as often as you can.
8. Make being active and eating healthier a family and friend affair *whenever possible.*
9. Put a note card on your refrigerator to remind yourself of habits you are trying to kick (e.g., No more sodas, No more *Oreos*, No more chips, No more eating after eight, etc.).
10. Manage stress/handle issues, and try to get at least six *plus* hours of sleep *every* night.

Would you believe that these ten steps can help you see dramatic results in a matter of months? Believe it or not, if you left everything else the same, these changes alone could make a huge difference in your weight! This is basically all I did in *Wake-up Call #3* (see Chapter 3) when I lost almost twenty pounds. I know changing a lot of things at once (e.g., having cereal/oatmeal instead of doughnuts for breakfast, water instead of soda, fruit in place of some snacks, etc.) can cause you to mentally shut down and cause your "*diet*" or "*get healthier*" efforts to fail within days. That's why I thought I would simplify things for anyone who wants a *get-started-quick* plan. So if everything else that you have heard so far has overwhelmed you, how about you just start with these ten steps over the next thirty days? Leave almost everything else the same as you adjust. Then after thirty days, check your progress, and make more changes as you are able. Continue to readjust/refine habits as needed, and I guarantee it will get easier.

You have nothing to lose but weight, *so why not try it?* Until you do, please don't move on to any other diet plan. *Be sure to give this "lifetime plan" 100 percent of your effort.* **This is your time to make it happen.** I wish you all the best as you work to reach and maintain your healthiest weight. As you do, stay strong and keep believing you can do it—*Because You Can!*

ᏽ

E p i l o g u e
· ~ · ~ · ~ ~ · ~ · ~ ·

"You have to work with what you've got. Don't judge what you have, just love it."
Anne Hathaway

The Devil Wears Prada is one of my favorite movies, but a conversation between one of the main characters and Anne Hathaway causes me a little mental distress from time to time… In the scene I am talking about, Anne is taking a little ribbing for the lunch she has chosen, and her companion lets her in on how the fashion industry views women's sizes (mainly hers)—*"…two became the new four, and zero became the new two."* If you saw the movie, you know this was not said nicely… However, Anne's character does try to come back by saying, *"Well, I'm a 6…"* At this point, most of us in the real world, who are not even a size 4, *much less a two or zero* are thinking this should be more than OK—*end of conversation, right?* WRONG!

The "friend" then delivers a parting, knockout punch, *"…which is the new fourteen."* Then for the rest of the movie he proceeds to call her *"6"* until she slims down to a size 4…. Of course I was happy for her, and she *did* look good, especially as her character had evolved during the movie. However, now occasionally when I say I am a size 6, I think of the line from the movie about it being *the new fourteen.* As a result, **now I wanna be a size 4 too!!!!!!** At times this desire created such a frenzy that I even looked into "shortcuts" such as liposuction or a tummy tuck. I know for a fact, if I ran more, I could be a size 4, but I am too lazy to run far or often, which is why cosmetic surgery seemed an "easier" (*albeit costly / risky*) alternative.

Shocking isn't it? Here I am, a mature woman, who is ordinarily pretty happy with her lot in life, but watching one movie (*albeit repeatedly*) was enough to undermine some of the self-esteem it took a lifetime to build… Needless to say when I came back to my senses, I realized that I am too big of a chicken to ever let someone poke a long, hot, metal tube quickly and roughly into my love handles or to cut off the excess skin from my stomach (*courtesy of my two sons*), pull it down, and sew me back together! *I am vain, but come on!* It grosses me out even to write about it, much less have it done! So if you ever see me, and I am a size 4, it will be because I ran more and ate less treats. Otherwise, I will just have to live with being a size 6 and just being able to fit into *my own* skinny jeans, not in someone else's (*e.g., Naomi Campbell's, Anne Hathaway's, Jada Pinkett-Smith's, etc.*). That's what makes me a skinny jean queen… *Being able to comfortably fit into my favorite pair of jeans and loving the way I look in them.* With that as the criteria, anyone can be a skinny jean queen if they choose to be. Do you want to be a skinny jean queen? If so, **just focus on the right size for *you* and work to fit / stay in *your own* skinny jeans.**

More About Carolyn Gray

Seminars, Conferences, and Speaking Engagements

Carolyn Gray offers dynamic and compelling workshops, seminars, boot camps, and talks in person for large and small groups, as well as via the Internet. Her webinars and live tele-seminars are a convenient way for you to gain insight and clarity on the habits/behaviors that have been preventing you from fitting into your favorite *"skinny jeans"* and reaching your long-term weight loss goals. She will help you experience your own personal wake-up call, and then motivate you to make changes. *To **do** something different. To **be** different. To **achieve** your goals.*

Personal Consultations

For those who wish to work in one-on-one sessions, Carolyn Gray also offers *Life-* and *Body-*Changing Consultations. These consultations are conducted by phone, via *Skype*, or in person and are designed to help you devise a lifetime plan that will not only get you in your "skinny jeans," but **keep you in them!** *Just like Carolyn did...* Sometimes you just need an objective ear to listen and then help you uncover what might be holding you back in your quest to lose the weight and keep it off. Carolyn's consultations provide that ear, as well as support and the *gentle/forceful* nudges (*whichever you need most at the time*) to help you achieve your goals. You will walk away from these powerful consultations with the tools you need to make life-changing breakthroughs and transformations where your weight *and* thinking are concerned. So what are you waiting for? *She's only a phone call away!*

Contact Information

If you would like to book Carolyn for an event or consultation, order books, or find out how to form an *Eat and Act Like You Have Some Sense* Support Group in your area, please visit her Web site:

www.CarolynGrayInternational.com

or contact her office at:

Carolyn Gray International, LLC
5746 Union Mill Road, PMB 495
Clifton, VA 20124
Phone: 703-830-2759
Email: info@CarolynGrayInternational.com
Carolyn@CarolynGrayInternational.com
Blogs: www.SecretsOfASkinnyJeanQueen.com
www.eFormationTonight.com
Twitter: www.twitter.com/eFormationQueen
YouTube: www.youtube.com/eFormationQueen

Carolyn would also love to hear your *Eat and Act Like You Have Some Sense* success story. Please send your stories to **Success@CarolynGrayInternational. com.**

.

Made in the USA
Lexington, KY
10 March 2010